Fast Facts

Vascular Surgery Highlights 2005–06

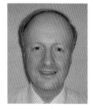

Edited by Alun H Davies MA DM FRCS
Reader and Honorary Consultant
Department of Vascular Surgery
Imperial College School of Medicine
Charing Cross Hospital, London, UK

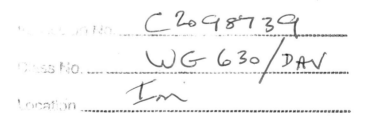
✝ HEALTH PRESS

Fast Facts: Vascular Surgery Highlights 2005–06
First published March 2006

© 2006 in this edition Health Press Limited
Health Press Limited, Elizabeth House, Queen Street, Abingdon,
Oxford OX14 3LN, UK
Tel: +44 (0)1235 523233
Fax: +44 (0)1235 523238

Book orders can be placed by telephone or via the website.
For regional distributors or to order via the website, please go to:
www.fastfacts.com
For telephone orders, please call 01752 202301 (UK), +44 1752 202301 (Europe),
1 800 247 6553 (USA, toll free) or +1 419 281 1802 (Americas).

Fast Facts is a trademark of Health Press Limited.

A CIP record for this title is available from the British Library.

ISBN 1-903734-83-5

Davies, AH (Alun)
Fast Facts: Vascular Surgery Highlights 2005–06/
Alun H Davies

Medical illustrations by Annamaria Dutto, Withernsea, UK.
Typesetting and page layout by Zed, Oxford, UK.
Printed by Fine Print (Services) Ltd, Oxford, UK.

Printed with vegetable inks on fully biodegradable and
recyclable paper manufactured from sustainable forests.

444   001
Low emissions
during production

Low
chlorine

Sustainable
forests

Introduction

Once more it is time for a new edition of *Fast Facts: Vascular Surgery Highlights*. The series has proved to be very popular, and I trust you will find this year's book as stimulating to read as previous editions. The topics are presented by experts in their field and range from the management of varicose veins to that of complicated aortic aneurysm repair.

Again I would like to thank the contributors and publishers for all their help in the production of this edition.

Alun H Davies MA DM FRCS
Reader and Honorary Consultant Surgeon
Department of Vascular Surgery
Imperial College School of Medicine
Charing Cross Hospital
London, UK

EVAR and DREAM trials for abdominal aortic aneurysm repair

Gaetano Deleo MD, Claudia Piazzoni MD, Valter Camesasca MD,
Alberto Froio MD, Angela Liloia MD, Maria Teresa Occhiuto MD,
Maria Rosa Piglionica MD and Giorgio Maria Biasi MD
Department of Surgical Sciences and Intensive Care,
University of Milan–Bicocca, Italy

Endovascular aneurysm repair (EVAR) of abdominal aortic aneurysms (AAA) is less invasive than open repair and can be used when the aortic anatomy is suitable; it appears to offer short-term benefits. Evidence from registries and trials is now available to guide the management of patients with AAAs.

EVAR registries

During the past 8 years, two large-scale multicenter registries have been started to monitor the results of EVAR: the European Collaborators' Registry on Stent–graft Techniques for Aortic Aneurysm Repair (EUROSTAR),[1] and the Registry for Endovascular Treatment of Aneurysms (RETA).[2] The data from these registries underline the need for long-term surveillance after EVAR. The 30-day mortality after EVAR is approximately 3%, and 25–40% of patients have complications that require additional interventions or conversion to open repair. Registries have the advantage of recruiting large numbers of patients (more than 7000 in EUROSTAR) with no restriction on methods and materials as in a trial protocol and no limitation to recruitment,[3] but randomized controlled trials are necessary to investigate the long-term results of EVAR.

The DREAM and EVAR trials

In 1999, the Dutch Randomised Endovascular Aneurysm Management (DREAM) trial and the UK EVAR trial 1 started

7

recruiting patients, with both following a similar protocol.[4–7] Initial results from these trials are now available.

The DREAM trial. Recruitment into this randomized, multicenter trial ended in 2002, with 153 patients receiving randomized treatment: 78 were treated with EVAR and 75 had conventional open repair.[8] The study patients were over 60 years old and had an AAA of at least 5 cm; they had to be fit enough for open and endovascular repair. Each participating center was required to have performed at least 30 conventional AAA repairs per year, and 50 endovascular procedures per year, and the referring surgeon and radiologist must have passed the learning curve and have carried out more than 20 endovascular procedures. Randomization was by telephone call from the randomization center.

The primary outcome was the combined perioperative mortality and morbidity. Quality of life (QoL) was assessed, using the Medical Outcomes Short-Form 36 (SF-36) instrument, the EuroQol Group's EQ-5D instrument and a questionnaire about sexual function. The two treatments were also compared in terms of cost effectiveness, with analysis of the costs of staff, investigations, drugs and overheads and costs per life-year gained.

The EVAR trials recruited patients with a minimum age of 60 and an AAA of more than 5.5 cm according to a computed tomographic (CT) scan. Patients fit for both endovascular and open repair were offered entry into EVAR trial 1, while patients unfit for open repair were entered into EVAR trial 2.[9] The primary endpoint for both trials was all-cause mortality.

The secondary outcomes of EVAR trial 1 were aneurysm-related mortality, the incidence of postoperative complications of aneurysm repair, re-interventions, QoL (measured with the SF-36 and EQ-5D instruments) and hospital costs.

EVAR trial 2 compared endovascular treatment with no intervention, based on the hypothesis that EVAR would reduce the risk of aneurysm-related death and improve long-term survival and QoL.

Thirteen eligible UK hospitals were chosen when they had completed 20 EVAR procedures. Randomization was stratified by center and done centrally by the trial manager.

Recruitment into EVAR trial 1 ended in 2003 – there were 1082 randomized patients, 543 of whom were assigned to the EVAR arm.[10] EVAR trial 2 recruited 338 patients: 166 patients were allocated to the EVAR arm with 172 patients in the 'no intervention' arm.[11]

Short-term results. The 30-day mortality in EVAR trial 1 was 4.7% in patients who had open repair compared with 1.7% in those who had EVAR.[12] In the DREAM trial, the number of patients was smaller, but the results were similar: 4.6% with open repair and 1.2% with EVAR.[8,13]

The EVAR trials included AAAs of diameter greater than 5.5 cm, while the DREAM trial enrolled AAAs over 5 cm in size, and, from EUROSTAR data, we know that aneurysm-related mortality after EVAR is higher in those with larger AAAs. Nevertheless, there is a convergence of data from the two trials showing a reduction in short-term mortality in those who have endovascular treatment.[14]

Longer-term results. Major concerns remain regarding the durability of EVAR and the need for costly and potentially complicated re-intervention.

In EVAR trial 1, the overall mortality at 4 years did not differ between patients in the EVAR group and those in the open repair group, while the aneurysm-related mortality was significantly different: 4% for EVAR compared with 7% for open repair ($p = 0.04$).[12] In the DREAM trial, the 1-year survival was 89% after open repair and 95% after EVAR, with an event-free survival of 72% in those who had open repair and 76% in the EVAR group.[13]

There were more late complications after EVAR than after open repair, and this has important implications for surveillance and costs. In EVAR trial 1, EVAR was associated with a 33% increase in hospital costs. The rate of re-intervention continues to increase

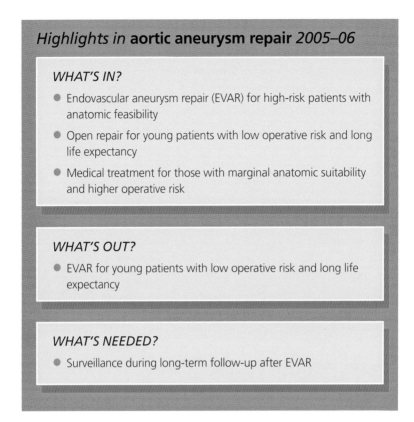

Highlights in **aortic aneurysm repair** 2005–06

WHAT'S IN?

- Endovascular aneurysm repair (EVAR) for high-risk patients with anatomic feasibility
- Open repair for young patients with low operative risk and long life expectancy
- Medical treatment for those with marginal anatomic suitability and higher operative risk

WHAT'S OUT?

- EVAR for young patients with low operative risk and long life expectancy

WHAT'S NEEDED?

- Surveillance during long-term follow-up after EVAR

yearly, so EVAR is more costly for patients with a long life expectancy, for whom open repair seems to be preferable.[10]

Quality of life analysis shows differences in data from the two trials. The DREAM trial reported deterioration in QoL after both EVAR and open repair, particularly in the first 3 weeks after the intervention; the decrease in QoL was most apparent in the patients who had had open repair, probably reflecting the more invasive nature of the procedure. By 3 months, both groups of patients had regained the preoperative levels of QoL, and at 1 year the QoL in the patients who had had open repair was significantly better than that in the EVAR group.[8] This is in contrast with the results of EVAR trial 1, which found no difference between the two groups at 3, 12 and 24 months.[12] In EVAR trial 2, with older patients, there was no QoL benefit for EVAR compared with no intervention; EVAR was associated with a 30-day operative mortality of 9% and a 4-year survival of 36%, with no difference in overall survival between the patients who had EVAR and the patients who received no intervention.[9] The results from EVAR trial 2 indicate that EVAR does not improve survival in patients with a short life expectancy and is not a safe procedure in high-risk patients, offering no survival benefit.

Effect on sexual function. A secondary aim of the DREAM trial was to assess sexual function in the first year after elective EVAR or open repair. An impact on sexual function was reported after both treatments, with a faster recovery to preoperative levels in patients who had EVAR than in those who had open repair; sexual function was similar in both groups at 3 months.[15]

References

1. Vallabhanemi SR, Harris PL. Lessons learnt from the EUROSTAR registry on endovascular repair of abdominal aortic aneurysm. *Eur J Radiol* 2001;39:34–41.

2. Thomas SM, Beard JD, Ireland M et al. on behalf of the Vascular Society of Great Britain and Ireland and the British Society of Interventional Radiology. Results from the Prospective Registry of Endovascular Treatment of Abdominal Aortic Aneurysms (RETA): mid-term results to five years. *Eur J Vasc Endovasc Surg* 2005;29:563–70.

3. Liapis CD, Kakisis JD. Value of registries for EVAR. *Eur J Vasc Endovasc Surg* 2005;30:341–2.

4. Prinssen M, Buskens E, Blanknsteijn JD. The Dutch Randomised Endovascular Aneurysm Management (DREAM) trial. Background, design and methods. *J Cardiovasc Surg* 2002;43:379–84.

5. Prinssen M, Verhoeven EL, Buth J et al. A randomized trial comparing conventional and endovascular repair of abdominal aortic aneurysms. *N Engl J Med* 2004;351:1607–18.

6. Brown LC, Epstein D, Manca A et al. The UK Endovascular Aneurysm Repair (EVAR) trials: design, methodology and progress. *Eur J Vasc Endovasc Surg* 2004;27:372–81.

7. EVAR trial participants. Endovascular aneurysm repair versus open repair in patients with abdominal aortic aneurysm (EVAR trial 1): randomised controlled trial. *Lancet* 2005;365:2179–86.

8. Prinssen M, Buskens E, Blanknsteijn JD on behalf of the DREAM trial participants. Quality of life after endovascular and open AAA repair. Results of a randomised trial. *Eur J Vasc Endovasc Surg* 2004;27:121–7.

9. EVAR trial participants. Endovascular aneurysm repair and outcome in patients unfit for open repair of abdominal aortic aneurysm (EVAR trial 2): randomised controlled trial. *Lancet* 2005;365:2187–92.

10. Cronenwett JL. Endovascular aneurysm repair: important mid-term results. *Lancet* 2005;365:2156–8.

11. www.evartrials.org

12. Greenhalgh RM, Brown LC, Kwong GP et al.; EVAR trial participants. Comparison of endovascular aneurysm repair with open repair in patients with abdominal aortic aneurysm (EVAR trial 1), 30-day operative mortality results: randomised controlled trial. *Lancet* 2004;364:843–8.

13. Blanknsteijn JD, De Jong SE, Prinssen M et al. Two-year outcomes after conventional or endovascular repair of abdominal aortic aneurysms. *N Engl J Med* 2005;352:2398–405.

14. Peppelenbosch N, Buth J, Harris PL et al. Diameter of abdominal aortic aneurysm and outcome of endovascular aneurysm repair: Does size matter? A report from EUROSTAR. *J Vasc Surg* 2004;39:288–97.

15. Prinssen M, Buskens E, Tutein Nolthenius RP et al. on behalf of the DREAM trial participants. Sexual dysfunction after conventional and endovascular AAA repair: results of the DREAM trial. *J Endovasc Ther* 2004;11:613–20.

Hybrid grafts for the management of thoracoabdominal aortic aneurysms

Robert E Brightwell BM MRCS(Eng) and
Nicholas JW Cheshire MD FRCS

Division of Surgery, Oncology, Reproductive Biology and Anaesthetics,
Imperial College London, and St Mary's Hospital, London, UK

A thoracoabdominal aortic aneurysm (TAAA) is defined by the involvement of the origins of the celiac, superior mesenteric and renal arteries. Crawford's classification system is universally accepted (Figure 1).[1]

TAAAs have high mortality and morbidity when treated by open techniques.[2,3] These risks persist despite advances in operative technique (including left heart bypass, spinal cord protection, hypothermic cardiopulmonary arrest, and selective visceral perfusion) and higher standards of perioperative care. The evolution of endovascular technology to treat infrarenal abdominal aortic aneurysms in the last 10 years has led to the possibility of treating TAAAs in this way.

The use of endovascular stents for the treatment of TAAA showed significant early promise, with several centers publishing encouraging results for endovascular stents. Use was limited to the thoracic segment because of the involvement of the origin of the visceral arteries.[4] Combining endovascular techniques with an open abdominal procedure has expanded the potential of endovascular therapy for TAAA. Such a 'hybrid' approach is attractive as it avoids thoracotomy, left heart bypass, extensive tissue dissection, excessive blood loss, and supraceliac aortic cross-clamp.

Early experience of visceral hybrid repair

A combined open and endovascular approach was first used to treat a TAAA in 1999 by Quinones-Baldrich et al.[5] In this instance, prior abdominal surgery and aneurysms of the visceral arteries precluded open repair. After this report, nine further individual cases/small

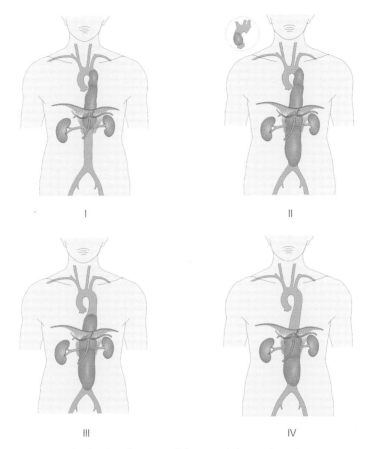

Figure 1 Crawford's classification of thoracoabdominal aortic aneurysms. Reproduced from Crawford et al. 1986[1] with permission from The Society for Vascular Surgery.

series using a hybrid approach in the treatment of TAAA were published.[6–14] The results of these individual cases were encouraging, despite the extremely complex nature of the disease and significant comorbidity of the patients being treated. It is worth highlighting that a non-standard technique was employed, and a variety of stent-grafts deployed.

Of the 20 patients reported in these series, only 1 (5%) died within a median follow-up period of 13 months. Spinal ischemia appeared to be rare (it was not reported in a single case), other complications were greatly reduced, and the length of stay in intensive care stay was reduced compared with open surgery.

Institutional technique of hybrid TAAA stent-grafting and visceral bypass

The patient is placed in a supine position under general and epidural anesthesia, with routine cerebrospinal fluid drainage. We routinely use cell salvage techniques (with rapid infusers available) and invasive monitoring with arterial and central venous lines, urethral catheterization, and transesophageal echocardiography.

A midline laparotomy allows for adequate exposure of the abdominal aorta, the origin of each renal artery, the celiac axis, and the superior mesenteric artery (SMA). The inflow site for visceral bypass grafting is determined by any previous abdominal aortic surgery and the distal extent of aneurysmal disease. Where a previous infrarenal repair has been undertaken, the bypass grafts are anastomosed in an end-to-side fashion to the existing graft. Where an infrarenal repair is possible, this is completed first, and bypass grafts are subsequently sutured as above. If the infrarenal aorta is normal, an arteriotomy is performed and the bypass grafts anastomosed in an end-to-side fashion to the native aorta: when aneurysmal disease extends to the bifurcation, one external iliac artery provides the inflow sites.

Most often, two inverted (14 × 7 mm or 16 × 8 mm) polyester grafts function as the conduits. The renal arteries are sequentially anastomosed in an end-to-side fashion. The two remaining graft limbs are routed along the base of the small bowel mesentery to the celiac axis and SMA in an end-to-side fashion. If Doppler signals are satisfactory in the bypass grafts (with the origins of the native vessel clamped) they are subsequently suture-ligated to prevent retrograde flow into the aneurysm sac (type II endoleak).

Following successful visceral and renal bypass, a suitable access site is chosen for endovascular stent deployment: usually a dedicated conduit attached to the common iliac artery or the abdominal aorta. An angiogram catheter is introduced on the contralateral side and the stents are deployed in a sequential fashion from the left subclavian artery through the thoracic aorta to the landing zone. Completion angiography after adjunctive procedures (extension cuff, balloon molding) then confirms exclusion of the aneurysm.

In our unit, we prefer this technique for Crawford type I, II, and III TAAAs, while an open approach with medial visceral rotation is used for Crawford type IV aneurysms.

Results of hybrid graft

Our results were presented at the 2005 meeting of the Society for Vascular Surgery, but up-to-date results are summarized in Table 1.[14]

Advantages of hybrid approach to TAAA

We perceive several advantages of this approach over standard open techniques.

- The technique avoids thoracotomy, so potentially there are fewer pulmonary complications and fewer cardiac arrhythmias, and patients have less pain.
- Hypothermia is reduced, with a subsequent reduction in coagulopathy and cardiovascular instability.
- There is a lower risk of spinal ischemia.
- Less blood is lost.
- Patients spend a shorter time in the intensive care unit and in hospital.
- More patients with comorbidities can be treated.

The future

The hybrid approach to TAAA may be a bridging measure until the technology of branched endovascular stent-grafts (EVSG) becomes established. Endovascular repair of juxtarenal and suprarenal abdominal aortic aneurysms with preservation of visceral perfusion by fenestrated[16,17] or branched[18] EVSG has been shown to be feasible and, using similar technology, several authors have described total endovascular repair of complex thoracic aortic disease.[19–20] Until recently, Chuter et al. were the only authors to report total endovascular repair of a TAAA with preservation of all

TABLE 1

Hybrid graft results from the Regional Vascular Unit, St Mary's Hospital, London, UK

- n = 34 patients
  - age: median 73 years, range 37–81 years
  - 25 elective, 6 urgent, 3 emergency
  - Crawford type I (4), type II (19), type III (10) and type IV (1)
- 31 (94%) had a completed procedure
- Mean ischemic time: 15 minutes (range 13–27 min) for each anastomosis
- No paraplegia within 30 days
- Elective mortality: 19%
- Endoleak: type I (8), type II (2), type III (1)
- Hospital stay: median 26 days, range 14–105 days
- 96.3% of visceral grafts were patent at median follow-up of 8 months

four visceral vessels in a single patient.[21] Anderson et al. reported a series of 4 patients treated in this way: 12 of 13 target vessels were revascularized, with no endoleaks. Three of the patients required further procedures to correct bleeding from access vessels, and 1 patient died from multi-organ dysfunction syndrome after such a procedure. Computed tomography at 12 months confirmed antegrade perfusion in all ten target vessels.[22]

Further improvement of, and access to, such devices, and correct patient selection (in light of the EVAR trial 2 results)[23] will see a reduction in the numbers of hybrid procedures being performed for TAAA. In the meantime, and in cases not suitable for repair using fenestrated/branched EVSG, the hybrid approach provides an adaptable and robust method of treating this complex disease.

Highlights in **hybrid grafts for the management of thoracoabdominal aortic aneurysms** *2005–06*

WHAT'S IN?

- A hybrid approach to thoracoabdominal aortic aneurysm (TAAA) in elective and emergency cases optimizing the use of stent-grafts

- An expanded population with complex TAAA can now be offered treatment

WHAT'S OUT?

- Universal open repair of TAAA

WHAT'S CONTROVERSIAL?

- Staged procedures

- Impact of fenestrated or branched endovascular stent-grafts

References

1. Crawford ES, Crawford JL, Safi HJ et al. Thoracoabdominal aortic aneurysms: preoperative and intraoperative factors determining immediate and long-term results of operations in 605 patients. *J Vasc Surg* 1986;3:389–404.

2. Svensson LG, Crawford ES, Hess KR et al. Experience with 1509 patients undergoing thoracoabdominal aortic operations. *J Vasc Surg* 1993;17:357–70.

3. Svensson LG, Crawford ES, Hess KR et al. Dissection of the aorta and dissecting aortic aneurysms: improving early and long-term surgical results. *Circulation* 1990; 82:IV24–38.

4. Dake MD, Miller DC, Mitchell RS et al. The "first generation" of endovascular stent-grafts for patients with aneurysms of the descending thoracic aorta. *J Thorac Cardiovasc Surg* 1998;111:689–703.

5. Quinones-Baldrich WJ, Panetta TF, Vescera CL et al. Repair of type IV thoracoabdominal aneurysm with a combined endovascular and surgical approach. *J Vasc Surg* 1999;30: 555–60.

6. Macierewicz JA, Jameel MM, Whitaker SC et al. Endovascular repair of perisplanchnic abdominal aortic aneurysm with visceral vessel transposition. *J Endovasc Ther* 2000;7:410–14.

7. Juvonen T, Biancari F, Ylönen K et al. Combined surgical and endovascular treatment of pseudoaneurysms of the visceral arteries and of the left iliac arteries after thoracoabdominal aortic surgery. *Eur J Vasc Endovasc Surg* 2001;22:275–7.

8. Watanabe Y, Ishimaru S, Kawaguchi S et al. Successful endografting with simultaneous visceral artery bypass grafting for severely calcified thoracoabdominal aortic aneurysm. *J Vasc Surg* 2002;35:397–9.

9. Khoury M. Endovascular repair of recurrent thoracoabdominal aortic aneurysm. *J Endovasc Ther* 2002;9:II106–11.

10. Agostinelli A, Saccani S, Budillon AM et al. Repair of coexistent infrarenal and thoracoabdominal aortic aneurysm: combined endovascular and open surgical procedure with visceral vessel relocation. *J Thorac Cardiovasc Surg* 2002;124:184–5.

11. Saccani S, Nicolini F, Beghi C et al. Thoracic aortic stents: a combined solution for complex cases. *Eur J Vasc Endovasc Surg* 2002;24: 423–7.

12. Fleck TM, Hutschala D, Tschernich H et al. Stent graft placement of the thoracoabdominal aorta in a patient with Marfan syndrome. *J Thorac Cardiovasc Surg* 2003;125:1541–3.

13. Rimmer J, Wolfe JHN. Type III thoracoabdominal aortic aneurysm repair: a combined surgical and endovascular approach. *Eur J Vasc Endovasc Surg* 2003;26:677–9.

14. Flye MW, Choi ET, Sanchez LA et al. Retrograde visceral vessel revascularisation followed by endovascular aneurysm exclusion as an alternative to open surgical repair of thoracoabdominal aortic aneurysm. *J Vasc Surg* 2004;39: 454–8.

15. Black SA, Wolfe JHN, Clark M et al. Complex thoraco-abdominal aortic aneurysms: endovascular exclusion with visceral revascularization. *Vascular Annual Meeting 2005, Chicago, IL, USA, Scientific program* 2005:abstr S16; 58.

16. Greenberg RK, Haulon S, O'Neill S et al. Primary endovascular repair of juxtarenal aneurysms with fenestrated endovascular grafting. *Eur J Vasc Endovasc Surg* 2004;27: 484–91.

17. Verhoeven ELG, Prins TR, Tielliu IFJ et al. Treatment of short-necked infrarenal aortic aneurysms with fenestrated stent-grafts: short-term results. *Eur J Vasc Endovasc Surg* 2004;27:477–83.

18. Hosokawa H, Iwase T, Sato M et al. Successful endovascular repair of juxtarenal and suprarenal aortic aneurysms with a branched stent graft. *J Vasc Surg* 2001;33:1087–92.

19. Inoue K, Iwase T, Sato M et al. Transluminal endovascular branched graft placement for a pseudoaneurysm: reconstruction of the descending thoracic aorta including the celiac axis. *J Thorac Cardiovasc Surg* 1997;114:859–61.

20. Bleyn J, Schol F, Vanhandenhove I et al. Side-branch modular endograft system for thoracoabdominal aortic aneurysm repair. *J Endovasc Ther* 2002;9:838–41.

21. Chuter TAM, Gordon RL, Reilly LM et al. An endovascular system for thoracoabdominal aortic aneurysm. *J Endovasc Ther* 2001;8:25–33.

22. Anderson JL, Adam DJ, Berce M et al. Repair of thoracoabdominal aneurysms with fenestrated and branched endovascular stent grafts. *J Vasc Surg* 2005;42:600–7.

23. Endovascular aneurysm repair and outcome in patients unfit for open repair of abdominal aortic aneurysm (EVAR trial 2): randomised controlled trial. *Lancet* 2005;365: 2187–92.

Spinal cord protection in thoraco-abdominal aortic aneurysm repair

Michael J Jacobs*† MD, Werner Mess‡ MD,
Geert Willem Schurink* MD and Gottfried Mommertz† MD

*Department of Vascular Surgery, University Hospital Maastricht,
The Netherlands; †Department of Vascular Surgery, University Hospital Aachen,
Germany; ‡Department of Neurophysiology, University Hospital Maastricht,
The Netherlands

During thoracoabdominal aortic aneurysm (TAAA) repair, spinal cord ischemia is likely to occur, followed by the devastating complication of paraplegia. In the most extensive aneurysms (type II) in particular, the paraplegia rate can be as high as 20%. Before the introduction of protective strategies, the speed of the operation was the main factor directly linked to the clinical outcome.

Several strategies for the preservation of spinal cord integrity have been developed during the last two decades. These adjunctive procedures include distal aortic perfusion,[1] cerebrospinal fluid (CSF) drainage[2,3] and systemic or local hypothermia.[4] Obviously, reattachment of intercostal and/or lumbar arteries is a prerequisite to re-establish the interrupted blood supply to the spinal cord.[5] A major impediment until recently, however, has been the inability to assess the efficacy of these protective strategies; the neurological outcome only becomes apparent after the patient wakes up. We could compare the process with flying a plane without a navigation system, which could likewise lead to unforeseen catastrophes. Thus, a reliable technique to assess spinal cord integrity during surgery is required.

Monitoring motor-evoked potentials (MEPs) is a technique that allows direct assessment of spinal cord function, dictating surgical strategies to restore and maintain blood supply to the gray matter.[6]

21

Distal aortic perfusion

During cross-clamping of the descending thoracic aorta, the intercostal and lumbar arteries are not perfused, leading to spinal cord ischemia. The simple but highly effective principle of distal aortic perfusion has improved the neurological outcome in patients undergoing TAAA repair. Distal aortic perfusion can be established by cannulation of the left atrium or pulmonary vein and the femoral artery. Alternatively, extracorporeal circulation can be implemented by means of femoral artery–vein cannulation. In a recent clinical study we have demonstrated the important role of lumbar arteries and the pelvic circulation in particular and its contribution to the collateral perfusion of the spinal cord.[7] Distal aortic perfusion is thus a highly valuable asset for spinal cord perfusion during aortic cross-clamping.

Cerebrospinal fluid drainage

During proximal cross-clamping of the descending thoracic aorta, CSF pressure increases significantly, compressing the small arteries that supply blood to the spinal cord. The rationale for the use of CSF drainage is to decrease CSF pressure to such a level that the pressure in the spinal-cord compartment no longer threatens the blood flow through the anterior spinal artery. Recently, a systematic review and meta-analysis addressed the effectiveness of CSF drainage to prevent neurological injury during TAAA repair.[8] All analyzed studies provided encouraging evidence that CSF drainage decreased paraplegia and lower-limb neurological deficits. The overall absolute risk reduction was 10%, indicating that only 10 patients must be treated with CSF drainage to prevent paraplegia in 1 patient. CSF drainage is also highly effective in patients developing delayed neurological deficits. Several reports and experiences have shown reversal of paraplegia by draining the CSF. The complication rate of the procedure itself, including subdural hematoma and meningitis, is lower than 1%. In our experience with more than 300 patients we have not encountered any complications of CSF drainage.

Reattachment of intercostal and lumbar arteries

In healthy subjects, approximately 26 intercostal and lumbar arteries between T5 and L5 contribute to spinal cord perfusion. The main radiculomedullary artery for the thoracolumbar spinal cord territory enters the vertebral canal between T9 and T12 in 75% of cases, between L1 and L3 in 10%, and between T5 and T8 in 15%.[9] In patients with degenerative TAAAs, the majority of these segmental arteries are occluded. In our experience, the median number of patent segmental arteries between T5 and L5 was only five.[7] Furthermore, in 16% of patients, the functional contribution to spinal cord blood supply mainly arose between L3 and L5, and in 8% of the patients it depended on the pelvic circulation. These findings illustrate the impressive collateral network that develops in patients with TAAAs.

Besides distal aortic perfusion, it is imperative to reattach the intercostal and lumbar arteries, especially in the area between T8 and L1.

Monitoring evoked potentials

The integrity of the spinal cord can be assessed intraoperatively using somatosensory-evoked potentials (SSEPs) or MEPs. A major drawback of SSEP monitoring is the occurrence of false-negative results, such as postoperative paraplegia despite unchanged SSEPs. This is because SSEPs assess conduction in the dorsal part of the spinal cord, whereas the motor neural system is located in the anterior horn.

Conduction in the anterior horn can be evaluated by means of MEP monitoring, the technique of which has been described in detail by Jacobs and Mess.[10] Basically, single MEPs are evoked to the scalp, and compound muscle action potentials are recorded from the skin over the left and right anterior tibialis muscle (Figure 1). As a reference, potentials are also recorded at the left and right thenar muscles.

Reduction of MEP amplitude at the anterior tibialis muscle during or after aortic cross-clamping indicates ischemic spinal cord dysfunction. On the basis of the MEP information, cord ischemia is

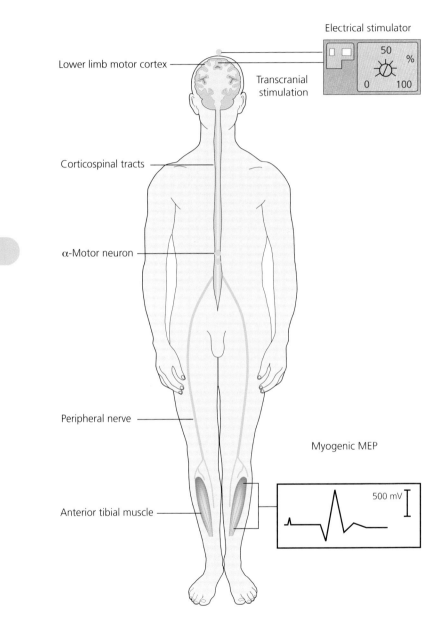

Electrical stimulator

Lower limb motor cortex

Transcranial stimulation

50 %

0   100

Corticospinal tracts

α-Motor neuron

Peripheral nerve

Myogenic MEP

Anterior tibial muscle

500 mV

Figure 1 Schematic representation of monitoring motor-evoked potentials.

corrected by means of several strategies. First, mean arterial pressure is increased, as well as distal aortic perfusion pressure, which will restore MEPs in the majority of patients.[7,11] Furthermore, MEP information guides selective reattachment of intercostal and/or lumbar arteries. Our principal achievement occurs when a certain segment of the aorta is cross-clamped and the MEPs disappear in the absence of a patent segmental artery. Without the MEP information, no further surgical actions would be considered and there is a high likelihood that the patient will wake up with paraplegia. In these circumstances, we perform aortic endarterectomy, which always provides back-bleeding arteries. These are subsequently revascularized by means of a short tube graft. In the majority of cases MEPs will be restored. If not, the patient will end up with a neurological deficit.

Using this modality over the last decade, we have been able to reduce the overall incidence of paraplegia to less than 3%.

The future

The surgical management of limited as well as extensive thoracic aortic aneurysms is gradually changing from maximally invasive repair to minimally invasive procedures in which endovascular and hybrid solutions, including side-branch technology, are increasingly important. However, extensive TAAAs still require open surgery, particularly in younger patients. Despite major improvements, morbidity and mortality remain high, especially in low-volume hospitals.[12] In addition to surgical expertise, patient outcome also depends greatly on the efforts of an integrated team consisting of high-level anesthesia, neuromonitoring, extracorporeal support, intensive care management and cardiology assistance. Infrastructure, team experience and dedication are the prerequisites for success. Therefore, TAAA repair should only be performed in centers meeting these criteria.

Highlights in **spinal cord protection in thoracoabdominal aortic aneurysm repair** *2005–06*

WHAT'S IN?

- Surgical protocol including distal aortic perfusion, reattachment of intercostal/lumbar arteries and drainage of cerebrospinal fluid

- Assessment of spinal cord function by monitoring motor-evoked potentials

- Thoracoabdominal aortic aneurysm (TAAA) repair only in specialized, high-volume centers

WHAT'S OUT?

- 'Clamp and go' technique

WHAT'S CONTROVERSIAL?

- Endovascular role in TAAA repair

WHAT'S NEEDED?

- Technical and material developments for endovascular procedures

- Preoperative anatomic and functional assessment of the spinal cord

References

1. Coselli JS, LeMaire SA. Left heart bypass reduces paraplegia rates after thoracoabdominal aortic aneurysm repair. *Ann Thorac Surg* 1999;67: 1931–4.

2. Safi HJ, Hess KR, Randel M et al. Cerebrospinal fluid drainage and distal aortic perfusion: reducing neurologic complications in repair of thoracoabdominal aortic aneurysm types I and II. *J Vasc Surg* 1996;23: 223–9.

3. Coselli JS, LeMaire SA, Koksoy C et al. Cerebrospinal fluid drainage reduces paraplegia after thoracoabdominal aortic aneurysm repair: results of a randomized clinical trial. *J Vasc Surg* 2002; 35:631–9.

4. Cambria RP, Darison K, Carter C et al. Epidural cooling for spinal cord protection during thoracoabdominal aneurysm repair: a five year experience. *J Vasc Surg* 2000; 31:1093–102.

5. Safi HJ, Miller CC, Carr C. Importance of intercostal artery reattachment during thoracoabdominal aortic aneurysm repair. *J Vasc Surg* 1998;27:58–68.

6. Jacobs MJ, Meylaerts SA, de Haan P et al. Strategies to prevent neurologic deficit based on motor evoked potentials in type I and II thoracoabdominal aortic aneurysm repair. *J Vasc Surg* 1999;29:48–59.

7. Jacobs MJ, de Mol BA, Elenbaas T et al. Spinal cord blood supply in patients with thoracoabdominal aortic aneurysms. *J Vasc Surg* 2002;35:30–7.

8. Cina CS, Abouzahr L, Arena GO et al. Cerebrospinal fluid drainage to prevent paraplegia during thoracic and thoracoabdominal aortic aneurysm surgery: a systematic review and metaanalysis. *J Vasc Surg* 2004;40:36–44.

9. Lazorthes G. Arterial vascularization of the spinal cord. Recent studies of the anastomatic substitution pathways. *J Neurosurg* 1971;35:253–62.

10. Jacobs MJ, Mess WH. The role of evoked potential monitoring in operative management of type I and II thoracoabdominal aortic aneurysms. *Sem Thorac Cardiovasc Surg* 2003;15:353–64.

11. Jacobs MJ, Mess W, Mochtar B et al. The value of motor evoked potentials in reducing paraplegia during thoracoabdominal aneurysm repair. *J Vasc Surg* 2006;42:239–46.

12. Cowan JA, Dimick JB, Henke PK et al. Surgical treatment of intact thoracoabdominal aortic aneurysms in the United States: hospital and surgeon volume-related outcomes. *J Vasc Surg* 2003;37:1169–74.

Ischemic complications of vascular access surgery

Marcus J Brooks MA MD FRCS (Gen Surg) and
Alun H Davies MA DM FRCS
Department of Vascular Surgery, Imperial College School of Medicine,
Charing Cross Hospital, London, UK

Hand and finger ischemia are important and often underrecognized complications of renal access surgery. Here we describe how a high preoperative index of suspicion for the presence of underlying arterial disease, routine duplex imaging and a preference for autologous vein fistula at the wrist will reduce the incidence of this complication. Care with fistula planning and creation is vital to identify pre-existing arterial stenoses and avoid arterial damage. No single test currently identifies the at-risk patient. It must be accepted that ischemia is often the consequence of a systemic process, not of the fistula itself.

The aim of management of established ischemia is to preserve both the limb and the access fistula. Percutaneous angioplasty or the distal revascularization and interval ligation (DRIL) procedure give the best results, as summarized below.

The evidence for interventions was collected from a Medline search using combinations of the following terms: renal access, ischemia, arm/*blood supply, hand/*blood supply, fingers/*blood supply, hemodialysis, vascular access and arteriovenous shunts.

Incidence

In the United Kingdom 37 per 100 000 of the population hemodialyse via an arteriovenous fistula or graft.[1] The year-on-year trend is for a 5% increase in this figure. The incidence of ischemic symptoms in this population is reported at between 6% and 20%, the higher percentage representing brachial artery fistulas and prosthetic grafts.[2–11] In a study of transposed autologous superficial femoral vein for brachial–axillary fistula the incidence of hand ischemia is even higher, at 43%.[12]

Pathophysiology

The principal causes of limb ischemia in patients with arteriovenous fistulas are large- and small-vessel occlusive arterial disease and the arterial steal phenomenon.

A fistula is a low-resistance shunt between the arterial and venous systems. Flow through the fistula is dependent on the arteriovenous pressure difference and fistula resistance, determined by the smallest diameter of the fistula. Typical flow rates for a radial–cephalic fistula are 500–800 mL/min, and for a brachial fistula 2000 mL/min. A flow rate of 50 mL/min is necessary to adequately perfuse the hand.[13,14] In studies of patients with upper-limb fistulas, 80–94% have been found to have retrograde arterial flow in the radial or ulnar arteries.[5,11] Since the majority of patients have no ischemic symptoms, it follows that the flow to the hand remains adequate.

A high proportion of patients with end-stage renal failure have atherosclerosis affecting medium and small arteries, including the palmar arch and digital arteries.[10] In most of these patients the disease is bilateral, diffuse and symmetrical. This may explain why patients who suffer ischemia are at increased risk when a new fistula is created in the contralateral limb: in a study of 23 patients with upper limb ischemia following a fistula, Yeager et al. found that 14 patients (61%) developed ischemia when a fistula was created in the contralateral limb.[10]

Symptoms and signs

The timing of onset of ischemia is variable, dependent on the progression of occlusive arterial disease, changes in fistula flow rates and the development of collaterals altering the dynamics of an arterial steal. Symptoms are often first manifested during dialysis when flow through the fistula increases. The diagnosis of ischemia can be clinically obvious for a threatened limb or cold hand with absent distal pulses that return as the fistula is compressed.

However, the diagnosis can be subtle and difficult to differentiate from diabetic neuropathy, sympathetic dystrophy or venous hypertension. Ischemic symptoms are occasionally confused with carpal tunnel syndrome.[15] In diabetic patients peripheral neuropathy may worsen with ischemia, and this condition, ischemic monomelic neuropathy, is difficult to treat, as symptoms may persist even once the limb has been successfully revascularized.

Degree of ischemia. The simple classification system shown in Table 1, a modification of the Fontaine classification for lower-limb ischemia, is used to define the degree of ischemia.

Predicting ischemia
No single preoperative test is sensitive and specific for the development of ischemia. A number of clinical risk factors have been identified:
- dialysis at a young age (< 55 years)
- diabetes mellitus
- coronary artery disease
- peripheral vascular disease.

The risk of arterial steal is higher with more proximal fistulas, high fistula flow rates and prosthetic grafts.[7–9] Digital palpation of the radial and ulnar arteries, Allen's test and hand-held Doppler examination are adequate assessment before creation of fistulas at the wrist. For brachial fistulas, lower-limb fistulas and tertiary procedures, the arteries should be formally imaged, a task most

TABLE 1

Classification of degree of ischemia

Class I	Limb pale/dusky and/or cold
Class II	Pain during exertion or hemodialysis
Class III	Pain at rest
Class IV	Tissue loss

simply achieved with arterial duplex scanning. Transcutaneous pO_2 measurement, digital plethysmography with oximetry and pulsed Doppler are currently research tools; they are not used routinely as there is no absolute preoperative level at which ischemia is inevitable.[4,16,17]

Surgical technique for fistula creation

The risk of ischemia is minimized if the most distal fistula possible is created using autologous vein with an end-to-side anastomosis. There should be no significant arterial stenosis proximal to the fistula, and an adequate supply to the hand from other arteries. Ehsan and colleagues suggest that this be achieved for brachial fistulas by performing the venous anastomosis onto either the radial or ulnar artery origin in preference to the distal brachial artery.[18] In the construction of the fistula it is important to avoid arterial trauma by gentle tissue dissection, minimal handling of the artery and the use of soft clamps, slings or occlusion catheters to control back-bleeding.

Managing ischemic complications

The aim of management is to preserve both access for hemodialysis and an intact limb. This necessitates prompt diagnosis before significant tissue loss or nerve damage has occurred and correct identification of the cause of the ischemia.

Normal fistula flow, no steal. These patients have a compromised upper limb arterial supply as a result of coexisting occlusive arterial disease or arterial injury at the time of fistula formation. Most such patients are diabetic. The key step to management is to identify the sites of all hemodynamically significant arterial stenoses using a combination of arterial duplex and magnetic resonance or conventional angiography. The best technique is dependent on institutional experience and on whether a proximal or distal lesion is suspected. We identify lesions using duplex ultrasonography and reserve conventional angiography for interventional procedures or confirmation of arterial anatomy prior to surgery.

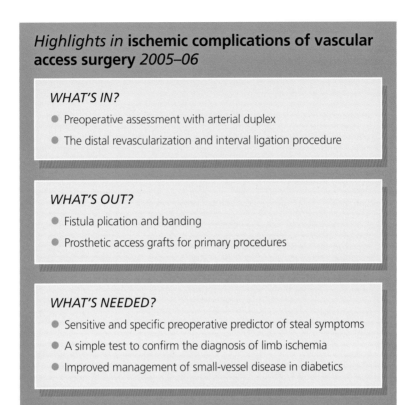

Highlights in **ischemic complications of vascular access surgery** *2005–06*

WHAT'S IN?

- Preoperative assessment with arterial duplex
- The distal revascularization and interval ligation procedure

WHAT'S OUT?

- Fistula plication and banding
- Prosthetic access grafts for primary procedures

WHAT'S NEEDED?

- Sensitive and specific preoperative predictor of steal symptoms
- A simple test to confirm the diagnosis of limb ischemia
- Improved management of small-vessel disease in diabetics

Proximal arterial stenoses are best treated by percutaneous angioplasty.[19,20] Modern guide wires and low-profile balloons mean that even distal upper-limb lesions are amenable to percutaneous intervention. The management of distal occlusive arterial disease is more difficult and may necessitate fistula ligation. A subsequent access procedure in the contralateral limb carries a high risk of ischemic complications.

Alternative options include grafts from the suprascapular or thoracic arteries, axillary–axillary interarterial chest-loop conduit, lower-limb access procedures, permacath insertion or even conversion to peritoneal dialysis.[21]

Arterial 'steal'. Steal from the palmar arch by a radial–cephalic fistula is cured by simple ligation of the artery distal to the fistula when the ulnar artery is patent. In some instances it is possible simply to ligate the distal artery even without a second supplying vessel.[7,22,23] When simple ligation is considered, it is prudent first to test the effect ligation will have using intra-arterial pressure monitoring. If collaterals alone are inadequate to supply the distal tissues, as with most brachial fistulas, simple ligation can be combined with a DRIL procedure, as described by Schanzer.[24] This technique adds resistance to retrograde arterial flow owing to the presence of two additional anastomoses and the jump graft itself. The DRIL procedure has been shown to improve both hemodynamic flow and the clinical state of the limb (Table 2).

The theoretical risk of the DRIL procedure is that thrombosis of the graft will result in acute limb ischemia. This complication has never been reported in the literature, presumably because of the development of a collateral circulation. Fistula plication, banding, interposition of a 4 mm poly(tetrafluoroethylene) bypass and the use of tapered grafts have all been used to increase resistance in the fistula and divert blood into the distal limb. These techniques have

TABLE 2

Distal revascularization and interval ligation procedure

Author	n	Relief from ischemia (%)	AVF patency (%)
Schanzer et al.[7]	14	93	82
Haimov et al.[25]	23	96	73
Katz et al.[26]	6	83	100
Berman et al.[2]	21	100	94
Lazarides et al.[27]	7	94	–
Stierli et al.[28]	6	100	100
Knox et al.[5]	52	90	83
Sessa et al.[29]	18	100	94
Diehl et al.[30]	14	100	71

AVF, arteriovenous fistula.

been largely abandoned, because once the band is applied tightly enough to reduce fistula flow significantly there is a high incidence of fistula thrombosis.[2,3]

Amputation or limb salvage. Class IV ischemia with tissue loss and necrosis may necessitate amputation of a finger or even the hand.[25,31,32] In all cases the fistula should be ligated or a DRIL procedure performed. One potentially useful technique for limb salvage with limited hand ischemia and a radial–cephalic fistula is to use a free flap anastomosed to the divided fistula.

References

1. Renal Registry, Southmead Hospital, Bristol BS10 5NB, UK: 2001.

2. Berman SS, Gentile AT, Glickman MH et al. Distal revascularization-interval ligation for limb salvage and maintenance of dialysis access in ischemic steal syndrome. *J Vasc Surg* 1997;26:393–402; discussion 402–4.

3. DeCaprio JD, Valentine RJ, Kakish HB et al. Steal syndrome complicating hemodialysis access. *Cardiovasc Surg* 1997;5:648–53.

4. Goff CD, Sato DT, Bloch PH et al. Steal syndrome complicating hemodialysis access procedures: can it be predicted? *Ann Vasc Surg* 2000;14:138–44.

5. Knox RC, Berman SS, Hughes JD et al. Distal revascularization–interval ligation: a durable and effective treatment for ischemic steal syndrome after hemodialysis access. *J Vasc Surg* 2002;36:250–5; discussion 256.

6. Morsy AH, Kulbaski M, Chen C et al. Incidence and characteristics of patients with hand ischemia after a hemodialysis access procedure. *J Surg Res* 1998;74:8–10.

7. Schanzer H, Skladany M, Haimov M. Treatment of angioaccess-induced ischemia by revascularization. *J Vasc Surg* 1992;16:861–4; discussion 864–6.

8. Wilson SE. Complications of vascular access procedures. In: Wilson SE, ed. *Vascular Access: Principles and Practice*, 4th edn. St Louis: Mosby, 2002:181–4.

9. Nicholson ML, Murphy GJ. Surgical considerations in vascular access. In: Conlon PJ, Schwab SJ, Nicholson ML, eds. *Haemodialysis Vascular Access: Practice and Problems*. Oxford: Oxford University Press, 2000:101–23.

10. Yeager RA, Moneta GL, Edwards JM et al. Relationship of hemodialysis access to finger gangrene in patients with end-stage renal disease. *J Vasc Surg* 2002;36:245–9; discussion 249.

11. Lazarides MK, Staramos DN, Panagopoulos GN et al. Indications for surgical treatment of angioaccess induced arterial steal. *J Am Coll Surg* 1998;187:422–6.

12. Huber TS, Hirneise CM, Lee WA et al. Outcome after autogenous brachial-axillary translocated superficial femoropopliteal vein hemodialysis access. *J Vasc Surg* 2004;40:311–18.

13. Wixon CL, Hughes JD, Mills JL. Understanding strategies for the treatment of ischemic steal syndrome after hemodialysis access. *J Am Coll Surg* 2000;191:301–10.

14. Wixon CL, Mills Sr. JL, Berman SS. Distal revascularization–interval ligation for maintenance of dialysis access and restoration of distal perfusion in ischemic steal syndrome. *Semin Vasc Surg* 2000;13:77–82.

15. Gousheh J, Iranpour A. Association between carpel tunnel syndrome and arteriovenous fistula in hemodialysis patients. *Plast Reconstr Surg* 2005;116:508–13.

16. Lin G, Kais H, Halpern Z et al. Pulse oxymetry evaluation of oxygen saturation in upper extremity with an arteriovenous fistula before and during hemodialysis. *Am J Kidney Dis* 1997;29:230–2.

17. Valentine RJ, Bouch CW, Scott DJ et al. Do preoperative finger pressures predict early arterial steal in hemodialysis access patients? A prospective analysis. *J Vasc Surg* 2002;36:351–6.

18. Ehsan O, Bhattacharya D, Darwish A et al. 'Extension technique': a modified technique for brachio–cephalic fistula to prevent dialysis access-associated steal syndrome. *Eur J Vasc Endovasc Surg* 2005;29:324–7.

19. Guerra A, Raynaud A, Beyssen B et al. Arterial percutaneous angioplasty in upper limbs with vascular access devices for haemodialysis. *Nephrol Dial Transplant* 2002;17:843–51.

20. Trerotola SO, Shah H, Johnson MS et al. Hemodialysis graft: use as access for upper and lower extremity arteriography and interventional procedures – initial experience. *Radiology* 1999;213:301–2.

21. Bünger CM, Kröger J, Kock L et al. Axillary–axillary interarterial chest loop conduit as an alternative for chronic hemodialysis access. *J Vasc Surg* 2005;42:290–5.

22. Balaji S, Evans JM, Roberts DE et al. Treatment of steal syndrome complicating a proximal arteriovenous bridge graft fistula by simple distal artery ligation without revascularization using intraoperative pressure measurements. *Ann Vasc Surg* 2003;17:320–2.

23. Chemla E, Raynaud A, Carreres T et al. Preoperative assessment of the efficacy of distal radial artery ligation in treatment of steal syndrome complicating access for hemodialysis. *Ann Vasc Surg* 1999;13:618–21.

24. Schanzer H, Schwartz M, Harrington E et al. Treatment of ischemia due to 'steal' by arteriovenous fistula with distal artery ligation and revascularization. *J Vasc Surg* 1988;7:770–3.

25. Haimov M, Schanzer H, Skladani M. Pathogenesis and management of upper-extremity ischemia following angioaccess surgery. *Blood Purif* 1996;14:350–4.

26. Katz S, Kohl RD. The treatment of hand ischemia by arterial ligation and upper extremity bypass after angioaccess surgery. *J Am Coll Surg* 1996;183:239–42.

27. Lazarides MK, Staramos DN, Kopadis G et al. Onset of arterial 'steal' following proximal angioaccess: immediate and delayed types. *Nephrol Dial Transplant* 2003;18:2387–90.

28. Stierli P, Blumberg A, Pfister J et al. Surgical treatment of steal syndrome induced by arteriovenous grafts for haemodialysis. *J Cardiovasc Surg (Torino)* 1998;39:441–3.

29. Sessa C, Riehl G, Porcu P et al. Treatment of hand ischemia following angioaccess surgery using the distal revascularization interval–ligation technique with preservation of vascular access: description of an 18-case series. *Ann Vasc Surg* 2004;18:685–94.

30. Diehl L, Johansen K, Watson J. Operative management of distal ischemia complicating upper extremity dialysis access. *Am J Surg* 2003;186:17–9.

31. Levine MP. The hemodialysis patient and hand amputation. *Am J Nephrol* 2001;21:498–501.

32. Nicholas JJ, Khanna P, Baldwin Jr D et al. Amputations associated with arteriovenous access. *Am J Phys Med Rehabil* 2000;79:180–3.

Management of vascular complications of drug abuse

Armando Mansilha MD PhD FEBVS and Sérgio Sampaio MD
Angiology and Vascular Surgery, Hospital de S João, Porto, Portugal

Drug abuse is a worldwide social concern, and drugs of abuse, such as amphetamines, cannabis, heroin and cocaine, are known to cause vascular damage.[1] Drug addiction, which entails vascular risks unknown to or misunderstood by physicians, now involves an increasing number of miscellaneous drugs, existing in manifold forms. Although the modern addict is skilled at achieving intravenous (IV) access, inexperience with sterile technique and lack of precise anatomic knowledge can lead to a number of complications associated with prolonged intravascular and perivascular injection of abused substances:

- ischemia following intra-arterial injection
- arterial and venous pseudoaneurysm
- vasculitis
- mycotic aneurysm
- aortic dissection
- abscess complicated by erosion of vessels
- arteriovenous fistula
- compartment syndrome
- superficial and deep-vein thrombosis (DVT)
- septic thrombophlebitis
- puffy hand syndrome.

Arterial injuries with ischemia

The first report of an accidental intra-arterial drug injection resulting in gangrene (in 1942) was the injection of pentothal sodium into an aberrant ulnar artery in a patient undergoing induction of general anaesthesia.[2] Whereas in earlier years, unintentional intra-arterial injections were primarily the action of physicians or nurses, now, most are associated with illicit drug use. This drug addiction is often accompanied by intercurrent pathologies that have their own vascular toxicity, particularly infection with human immunodeficiency virus (HIV). Moreover, clinical presentations are made still more complex by the advent of new illicit substances. The pathophysiological mechanisms involved are interwoven and complicated by the frequent association with polytoxicomania or by the effects of the excipients added to such drugs. These effects include direct vascular toxicity with spasm and endothelial damage, angiitis and arterial and venous thrombosis.[3]

There is no way to determine accurately the incidence of arterial injections associated with drug abuse or to describe fully the variety of resulting vascular insufficiency syndromes. Only the worst complications of intra-arterial drug injection come to medical attention, and it is possible that many inadvertent intra-arterial injections go unnoticed. Delay in seeking medical attention is common. It is possible for digital or even total extremity gangrene to be the presenting complaint. Intra-arterial drug injection may result in a fulminant syndrome of acute limb ischemia involving small vessels, and can progress to distal gangrene and tissue loss. The most common sites of intra-arterial injection are the radial and brachial arteries.

Cannabis is by far the most frequently consumed illicit psychoactive substance among 15–25-year-olds and may eventually provoke arterial disease similar to that found in thromboangiitis obliterans.[4] Cessation of cannabis smoking appears to have a favorable effect on ischemic symptoms.[5]

Cocaine abuse, including alkaloidal ('crack') cocaine, alone or in combination with tobacco, may cause a variety of vascular problems, including venous thrombosis, lower extremity vasospasm, mesenteric artery thrombosis, renal infarction and aortic dissection.[6] Although most lesions are inflammatory in nature, accelerated atherosclerosis has been reported.[7]

The long-term abuse of amphetamine derivatives such as 'speed' and 'ecstasy' also appears to play a role in the development of peripheral arterial occlusions and seems to have broad similarities with Buerger's disease.[8]

Management. Treatment of these arterial complications is frequently non-specific and should be aggressive. Medical management consists of supportive care with heparin anticoagulation to prevent further thrombosis, IV hydration to prevent renal failure from rhabdomyolysis if associated, analgesia, local skin care and measures to prevent local limb and systemic hypothermia. Development of compartment hypertension mandates fasciotomy. Thrombolysis is rarely used. Vasodilators may be used but are unlikely to be of benefit. Steroids like dexamethasone can be used to protect cellular integrity, limit edema and to control the release of inflammatory mediators in response to tissue ischemia.

Vascular reconstruction depends on the extension and localization of the lesion. When the distal arterial bed is occluded and symptoms of pain, coldness and ischemia are present, sympathectomy may be useful.

Mycotic aneurysm

Arterial mycotic aneurysm associated with drug injection results from repetitive needle trauma of the artery, along with bacterial inoculation of the area surrounding the vessel. The arterial wall may become aneurismal without direct needle trauma if infection extends from an adjacent site or if bacterial emboli from a distant site lodge in the vasa vasorum of the vessel wall and cause destruction.[9] Complications of mycotic aneurysm include rupture, thrombosis and distal embolization.

Treatment includes parenteral antibiotics, wide debridement of all infected tissue, proximal and distal ligation of the aneurysmal vessel and removal of the entire infected arterial segment. Immediate revascularization for acute ischemia is not necessary in many patients. Autogenous graft material is rarely available in these patients if revascularization needs to be done immediately. Furthermore, use of prosthetic grafts in these circumstances is associated with an increased risk of graft infection and occlusion, so the grafts should be routed through extra-anatomic, non-infected tissue planes.[10]

One of the most frequent vascular complications in drug addicts is the occurrence of infected pseudoaneurysms of the femoral, brachial or radial arteries. Surgical repair requires debridement, ligation and resection of the aneurysm, with revascularization, similar to that described above for mycotic aneurysms.[11]

Venous injuries

Venous damage associated with drug injection is usually the result of chronic or repetitive trauma producing local irritation of the venous endothelium, which can lead to thrombosis. This process most frequently involves the superficial extremity veins but may extend into the deep venous system. Occasionally, injections are made directly into the femoral veins. DVT resulting from repetitive IV drug injection is treated with anticoagulation, as with DVT resulting from any other cause. If septic thrombophlebitis is suspected, antibiotics are added to the regimen. *Staphylococcus aureus* is the organism most commonly isolated in these cases. Septic thrombophlebitis that does not respond to anticoagulation and antibiotic therapy requires surgical thrombectomy or vein excision. The common femoral vein may become pseudoaneurysmal after repeated injection, as with an arterial mycotic aneurysm. Treatment can be complete excision of the affected vein, with proximal and distal ligation.

Vascular access

Vascular access in IV drug abusers may become compromised by the repeated injection of toxic substances. In such circumstances, abusers are driven by their addiction to seek alternative routes of drug delivery. For example, chronic ulcers can be cultivated and maintained for the administration of heroin. In these cases, the patient's desire for wound healing may be overridden by their addiction. Successful treatment of these wounds therefore depends on cessation of drug abuse and patient compliance, which are most easily achieved with multidisciplinary care.[12]

Highlights *in* management of vascular complications of drug abuse *2005–06*

WHAT'S IN?

- Understanding of the gravity of different vascular injuries provoked by drugs of abuse

WHAT'S OUT?

- Immediate revascularization in any patient with acute ischemia

WHAT'S CONTROVERSIAL?

- Type of revascularization for ischemia
- Type of hemodialysis access in active intravenous (IV) drug abusers if fistula is not feasible

WHAT'S NEEDED?

- Dedicated psychiatric rehabilitation to prevent further IV drug abuse

Another important problem to be considered is the influence of IV drug abuse on access-placement practices for hemodialysis and access survival in HIV-infected patients.[13] Fistulas are the first choice for hemodialysis access in HIV-seropositive patients, regardless of the patient's history in terms of IV drug abuse. If this is not feasible, graft placement in non-users or abstinent IV drug abusers is recommended. The optimal method of renal replacement therapy and type of hemodialysis access for active IV drug users remains uncertain.

References

1. Sheperd RF, Rooke T. Uncommon arteriopathies: what the vascular surgeon needs to know. *Semin Vasc Surg* 2003;16:240–51.

2. Van der Post CWH. A case of mistaken injection of pentothal sodium into an aberrant ulnar artery. *S Afr Med J* 1942;16:182.

3. Vandhuick O, Pistorius MA, Jousse S et al. Drug addiction and cardiovascular pathologies. *J Mal Vasc* 2004;29:243–8.

4. Karila L, Danel T, Coscas S et al. Progressive cannabis-induced arteritis: a clinical thromboangiitis obliterans sub-group? *Presse Med* 2004;33:21–3.

5. Scheltinga MR, van der Geer S, Hauben E et al. Cannabis use and untreated HIV-infection: unknown risk factors for premature peripheral artery disease. *Ned Tijdschr Geneeskd* 2004;148:2403–8.

6. Swalwell CI, Davis GG. Methamphetamine as a risk factor for acute aortic dissection. *J Forens Sci* 1999;44:23–6.

7. Bacharach JM, Colville DS, Lie JT. Accelerated atherosclerosis, aneurysmal disease, and aortitis: possible pathogenetic association with cocaine abuse. *Int Angiol* 1992;11:83–6.

8. Leithauser B, Langheinrich AC, Rau WS et al. A 22-year-old woman with lower limb arteriopathy. Buerger's disease, or methamphetamine- or cannabis-induced arteritis? *Heart Vessels* 2005;20:39–43.

9. Chu PH, She HC, Lim KE, Chu JJ. Mycotic aneurysm of the superior mesenteric artery in a young woman. *Int J Clin Pract* 2005;59: 614–16.

10. Cheema MA, Shafique A. Presentation and management of pseudoaneurysms of femoral artery. *J Coll Phys Surg Pak* 2005;15:162–4.

11. Siu WT, Yau KK, Cheung HY et al. Management of brachial artery pseudoaneurysms secondary to drug abuse. *Ann Vasc Surg* 2005;19: 657–61.

12. Williams AM, Southern SJ. Conflicts in the treatment of chronic ulcers in drug addicts – case series and discussion. *Br J Plast Surg* 2005;58:997–9.

13. Eustace JA, Gregory PC, Krishnan M et al. Influence of intravenous drug abuse on vascular access placement and survival in HIV-seropositive patients. *Nephron Clin Pract* 2005;100:c38–45.

Renal artery stenosis

Rachel Abela MD FRCS and George Hamilton MD FRCS

Vascular Unit, University Department of Surgery, Royal Free and University College School of Medicine, University College London, London, UK

The first case of hypertension cured by surgical revascularization was reported in 1954.[1] After balloon angioplasty in 1978 came the Palmaz stent in the early 1990s, greatly broadening the potential to treat renal artery stenosis (RAS), a condition traditionally regarded as a correctable cause of hypertension and renal insufficiency. Unfortunately, however, it also led to a high rate of indiscriminate revascularization of incidental RAS, which is discovered in 47–50% of imaging procedures performed in the investigation of other central and peripheral vascular disease.[2,3] A deluge of conflicting data was subsequently generated, with various centers trying to champion their preferred modality of intervention.

Epidemiology and pathophysiology

The significance of RAS is its contribution – or otherwise – to renovascular hypertension, renal dysfunction and, ultimately, cardiovascular compromise and death. Atherosclerosis is the main cause of RAS in the West, accounting for 90% of cases. Fibromuscular dysplasia (FMD) is the second most common cause, mainly affecting young adults. The predominance of atherosclerosis reflects a progressive systemic condition in an aging population. In fact, although only 1–5% of all patients with hypertension have renovascular hypertension, up to 6.8% of the general population over 65 years old were found to have RAS of 60% or more.[4] In addition, RAS was found to progress at an average rate of 7% per year, with stenoses of over 60% progressing by 30% at 1 year and 48% at 3 years.[5] Unfortunately, there is no simple proportionate relationship between RAS, hypertension and renal dysfunction. Discounting prior insults to renal function caused by other renal and systemic disease, both renal hypoperfusion and hypertension in atherosclerotic RAS cause variable degrees of parenchymal damage and renal dysfunction, now known as atherosclerotic nephropathy. In addition, an initially reversible response by the renin–angiotensin–aldosterone system develops, after an unpredictable period of time, into a state of chronic renin secretion, sustained hypertension and fluid volume expansion. This complex interrelationship of events presents the main challenge in the choice and timing of treatment for patients with RAS.

Presentation and investigation

Clinically significant RAS is usually associated with one or more of the manifestations listed in Table 1. Suspicion of RAS associated with one or more of these manifestations should trigger further evaluation along two main directions.

TABLE 1

Clinical manifestations associated with renal artery stenosis

Hypertension

- Rapid-onset hypertension
- Accelerated hypertension
- Refractory hypertension
- Hypertension in childhood or young adulthood

Renal

- Sudden unexplained deterioration in renal function
- Deterioration in renal function related to ACE inhibitors or angiotensin-receptor blockers
- Unexplained hypokalemia/secondary hyperaldosteronism
- Unilateral shrunken kidney

Other

- Flash pulmonary edema and/or unexplained CHF
- Other atherosclerotic vascular disease

ACE, angiotension-converting enzyme; CHF, congestive heart failure.

- First, stenosis has to be diagnosed, localized and measured, and the individual's renal function should be assessed (Table 2).
- Secondary assessment should indicate whether treatment of the stenosis would contribute to the management of the patient's clinical problems.

The diagnosis of RAS previously depended on contrast angiography, with its associated hazards, which can be reduced by the use of carbon dioxide as a contrast agent. Recent advances in non-invasive imaging modalities allow assessment of renal arteries even in patients with reduced renal function. Spiral computed tomography angiography avoids catheterization but requires a similar contrast load. Magnetic resonance angiography has improved rapidly and, combined with phase-contrast flow, has been shown to have high interobserver agreement and also high intermodality agreement with digital subtraction angiography (97% of cases[6]); however, the need for enhancement by gadolinium, which is relatively nephrotoxic, is still a limiting factor. Duplex ultrasonography (sensitivity 84–98%; specificity 62–99%[7]), the only non-invasive imaging tool, assesses stenosis from the renal artery flow acceleration index. Although its

TABLE 2

An algorithm for investigation of renal function

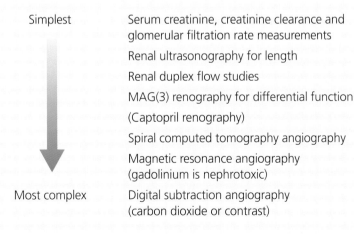

Simplest	Serum creatinine, creatinine clearance and glomerular filtration rate measurements
	Renal ultrasonography for length
	Renal duplex flow studies
	MAG(3) renography for differential function (Captopril renography)
	Spiral computed tomography angiography
	Magnetic resonance angiography (gadolinium is nephrotoxic)
Most complex	Digital subtraction angiography (carbon dioxide or contrast)

MAG(3), ^{99m}Tc-mercaptoacetyl triglycine.

use may be limited by patient habitus and operator dependency, it can be used to assess features that indicate renal function, such as renal size, cortical thickness and renal resistance index.[8]

Split renal function and glomerular filtration rate are also inferred from renal perfusion in scintigraphy studies such as MAG(3) (^{99m}Tc-mercaptoacetyl triglycine) renography. Scintigraphy can be supplemented by captopril challenge; however, this does not provide an accurate diagnosis of renovascular hypertension, except possibly in high-grade stenosis (> 80%).

Other tools to assess renal function include measurement of creatinine levels, creatinine clearance and the presence and extent of proteinuria. The severity of histopathological damage is an important determinant of renal function,[9] but renal biopsies have not yet found a place in the work-up of RAS because of the associated risk.

Management

Priorities in the management of RAS are the control of hypertension and optimization of renal function, with the expected benefit of improving cardiovascular morbidity and avoiding progression to dialysis-dependent renal failure. Most revascularization studies have shown that although a modest proportion of patients (25–30%) experience improved renal function, a significant proportion were stabilized or showed no benefit; indeed 19–25% had deteriorated function.[10] The angiogram in Figure 1 shows why revascularization

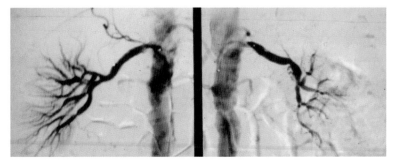

Figure 1 These selective renal angiograms demonstrate extensive segmental arteriosclerosis beyond the main renal artery stenosis.

of the main renal artery can fail. Other studies found that interventional treatment of RAS had little advantage over conservative management of renovascular hypertension, conferring only a modest reduction in antihypertensive medication.[11] A recent related study concluded that such a reduction did not lead to a detectable improvement in quality of life,[12] although long-term outcomes were not addressed.

Conservative management of renovascular hypertension includes:
- antihypertensive agents
- treatment of comorbid disease
- lipid-lowering agents
- antiplatelet agents
- lifestyle modifications (e.g. smoking cessation, weight loss).

The introduction of angiotension-converting enzyme (ACE) inhibitors in the early 1980s revolutionized the management of renovascular hypertension, increasing the rate of control from less than 50% to 82–96%.[13] ACE inhibitors and angiotensin-receptor blockers are known to reduce mortality in coronary disease and congestive heart failure, although they have caused deterioration in renal function in up to 6% of patients. Restoring the ability to use these agents has been proposed as an appropriate indication for revascularization.[10,14]

Revascularization. The indications for revascularization are summarized in Table 3. These need to be considered in the context of the patient's comorbidities and other recognized predictors of outcome. Positive predictors include:
- acute presentation/deterioration
- preserved left ventricular function[15]
- renal size greater than 8 cm
- serum creatinine concentration below 350 µmol/L
- renal resistance index below 808
- a single functioning kidney
- presence of a collateral blood supply with preserved cortical thickness.

Revascularization options include endovascular and open surgical

TABLE 3

Indications for revascularization in renal artery stenosis

- Deterioration in renal function and/or hypertension control despite maximum conservative treatment
- Flash or recurrent pulmonary edema and unstable angina (cardiac disturbance syndrome)
- Recent- or rapid-onset end-stage renal failure – 'salvage therapy'
- Acute renal failure in patients with cardiac disease while taking ACE inhibitors/angiotensin-receptor blockers
- Loss of renal mass on conservative treatment
- Progression of stenosis

ACE, angiotension-converting enzyme.

procedures. In RAS caused by FMD, angioplasty, with or without stenting, has consistently been shown to be the approach of choice, with surgery being indicated only for branch/segmental disease or in cases of endovascular failure requiring salvage. In atherosclerotic RAS, endovascular treatment (stent angioplasty) currently predominates (Figure 2). It is perceived to be a less invasive and cheaper option, with lower procedure-related morbidity and mortality than surgery. It is thus considered a useful option when surgery is contraindicated. Unfortunately, however, because of the ease of stent angioplasty, it is increasingly being used to

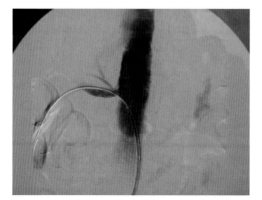

Figure 2 Stent angioplasty of a severe osteal renal artery stenosis.

revascularize RAS of disputable clinical significance detected incidentally during coronary and other angiography.[16] Many of the existing published findings concentrate on the technical and short-term success of angioplasty and stenting and imply that it is equivalent in efficacy to surgery, with lower morbidity and mortality, and is therefore preferable to surgery. In reality, the only objective comparisons that can be drawn between endovascular and open revascularization are cost and primary and secondary patency rates. Recently there has been interest in distal protection devices similar to those used in carotid angioplasty, but there is currently little evidence for clinical benefit.

Only patients with RAS that is causing significant clinical compromise are selected for surgery; this, together with the systemic nature of atherosclerotic disease, means that the surgical data are likely to include patients with higher risk factors. It is also not relevant to compare morbidity of percutaneous stenting of a single stenosed renal artery and open revascularization with that of concomitant aneurysm repair (Figure 3), although in dedicated

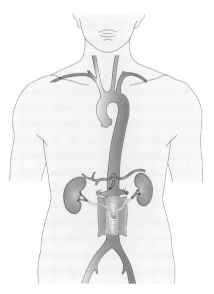

Figure 3 Combined resection of an abdominal aortic aneurysm and bilateral renal revascularization.

TABLE 4

Surgical revascularization options

- Aortorenal bypass (saphenous vein, PTFE, polyester)
- Aortic replacement with renal bypass
- Endarterectomy +/– patch closure
- Extra-anatomic native artery revascularization: hepatorenal (Figure 4), splenorenal, mesenterorenal
- Extra-anatomic bypass using saphenous vein or PTFE (from right hepatic or iliac arteries or supraceliac aorta)
- Bench reconstruction and autotransplantation (Figure 5)
- Nephrectomy

PTFE, poly(tetrafluoroethylene).

centers mortality has been found to be as low as 2.3%.[17] Five-year primary patency rates are higher for surgery (83–92%[18]) than for endovascular procedures, and mortality over 5 years is similar.[19] Furthermore, surgery offers a variety of procedural options (Table 4). Special considerations for the selection of surgery[20] are listed below:

- need for concomitant intervention for aortic aneurysm or stenosis
- segmental fibromuscular dysplasia (Figure 6)
- RAS > 2 cm (Figure 6)
- renal artery diameter of 4 mm or less
- severe ulcerative and unstable aortic atheroma
- long, diffuse renal artery lesions
- segmental disease
- renal artery occlusion
- contrast nephropathy
- lack of access for endovascular procedures
- salvage of failed endovascular procedures.

Pediatric renovascular disease (middle aortic syndrome, William's syndrome, neurofibromatosis, etc.) can be temporarily treated by angioplasty but usually requires surgical revascularization.

(a)

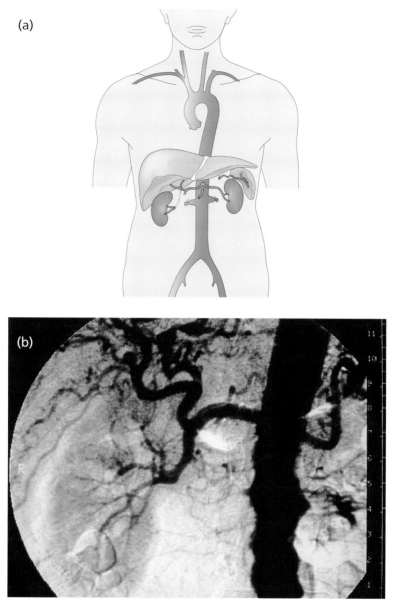

Figure 4 Extra-anatomic bypass for renal artery stenosis: (a) the hepatorenal bypass can be performed using the gastroduodenal artery which is of sufficient caliber in up to 40% of patients; (b) an angiogram showing a hepatorenal bypass 1 year after surgery.

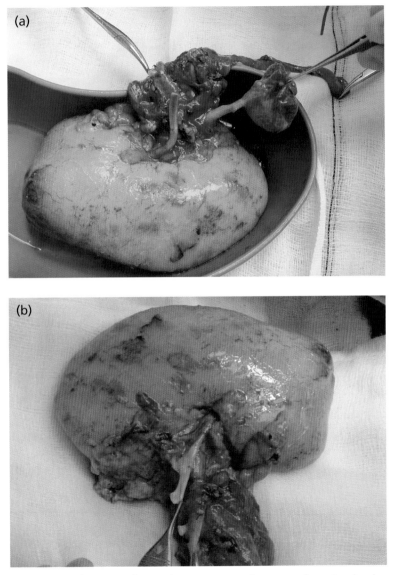

Figure 5 Bench surgery for renal aneurysm causing severe hypertension in a 16-year-old girl. (a) Extracorporeal repair of the renal aneurysm was performed in the left kidney prepared as for renal harvest and maintained in ice-cold saline. (b) An unhurried resection of the aneurysm from the cooled kidney was possible with reconstruction of the hilar arteries and autotransplantation into the left pelvis.

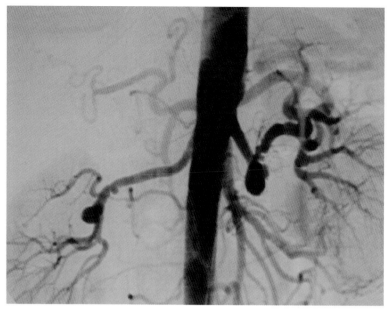

Figure 6 Segmental fibromuscular dysplasia and renal artery aneurysms greater than 2 cm in diameter remain indications for surgical repair.

Future trends

Many questions relating to the management of RAS remain unresolved, with few sufficiently powered randomized controlled trials and many conflicting results. Three ongoing trials are currently comparing the medical and endovascular management of RAS:

- ASTRAL: Angioplasty or Stent for Renal Artery Lesions
- STAR: Stenting in Renal Dysfunction Caused by Renal Artery Stenosis
- CORAL: Cardiovascular Outcomes in Renal Atherosclerotic Lesions.

The ASTRAL trial is by far the largest of these trials, aiming to recruit 1000 patients. The outcome seems highly likely to be the intriguing possibility that modern best medical management is all that is needed to treat the majority of patients with atherosclerotic renovascular disease. Revascularization will probably be limited to a minority of patients with specific indications, such as flash

53

Highlights in **renal artery stenosis** *2005–06*

WHAT'S IN?

- Magnetic resonance angiography, carbon dioxide angiography and spiral computed tomography angiography as preferred imaging techniques
- Vigilant use of best medical therapy as primary management
- Revascularization only if definitely indicated

WHAT'S OUT?

- Captopril renography for assessment of renal function
- Simple renal angioplasty

WHAT'S AWAITED?

- Results of the ASTRAL trial (over two-thirds of recruitment achieved to date)

pulmonary edema, ACE-inhibitor-induced renal failure or failed medical therapy. Surgical revascularization undoubtedly provides superior long-term results, but the probable higher mortality associated with this treatment means that it is justified only in the young and for fitter patients with atherosclerosis. A prospective randomized comparison of stent angioplasty and surgery would be of great value in providing evidence for management of these patients but is now unlikely ever to happen because of the small numbers of surgical procedures and reduced availability of surgical expertise. Thus, selection of patients for endovascular or vascular revascularization should depend on patient fitness but will more probably be based on the balance of endovascular and surgical skills available at individual centers.

References

1. Freeman N. Thrombend-arterectomy for hypertension due to renal artery occlusion. *JAMA* 1954;157:1077.

2. Rihal CS, Textor SC, Breen JF et al. Incidental renal artery stenosis among a prospective cohort of hypertensive patients undergoing coronary angiography. *Mayo Clin Proc* 2002;77:309–16.

3. Pillay WR, Kan YM, Crinnion JN, Wolfe JH; Joint Vascular Research Group, UK. Prospective multicentre study of the natural history of atherosclerotic renal artery stenosis in patients with peripheral vascular disease. *Br J Surg* 2002;89:737–40.

4. Hansen KJ, Edwards MS, Craven TE et al. Prevalence of renovascular disease in the elderly: a population based study. *J Vasc Surg* 2002;36:443–51.

5. Zierler RE, Berghelin RO, Davidson RC et al. A prospective study of disease progression in patients with atherosclerotic renal artery stenosis. *Am J Hypertens* 1999;12:1–7.

6. Schoenberg SO, Knopp MV, Londy F et al. Morphologic and functional magnetic resonance imaging of renal artery stenosis: a multireader tricenter study. *J Am Soc Nephrol* 2002;13:158–69.

7. Carman T, Olin JW, Czum J. Noninvasive imaging of renal arteries. *Urol Clin North Am* 2001;28:815–26.

8. Radermacher J, Chavan A, Bleck J et al. Use of Doppler ultrasonography to predict the outcome of therapy for renal artery stenosis. *N Engl J Med* 2001;344:410–17.

9. Wright JR, Duggal A, Renu T et al. Clinicopathological correlation in biopsy-proven atherosclerotic nephropathy: implications for renal functional outcome in atherosclerotic renovascular disease. *Nephrol Dial Transplant* 2001;16:765–70.

10. Textor SC. Ischemic nephropathy: where are we now? *J Am Soc Nephrol* 2004;15:1974–82.

11. van Jaarsfeld BC, Krijnen P, Pieterman H et al. The effect of balloon angioplasty on hypertension in atherosclerotic renal artery stenosis. *N Engl J Med* 2000;342:1007–14.

12. Krijnen P, van Jaarsfeld BC, Hunink M et al. The effect of treatment on health-related quality of life in patients with hypertension and renal artery stenosis. *J Hum Hypertens* 2005;19:467–70.

13. Textor SC. ACE inhibitors in renovascular hypertension. *Cardiovasc Drugs Ther* 1990;4:229–35.

14. Main J. Atherosclerotic renal artery stenosis, ACE inhibitors and avoiding cardiovascular death. *Heart* 2005;91:548–52.

15. Zeller T, Frank U, Müller C et al. Predictors of improved renal function after percutaneous stent-supported angioplasty of severe atherosclerotic ostial renal artery stenosis. *Circulation* 2003;108:2244–9.

16. Textor SC. Atherosclerotic renal artery stenosis: how big is the problem and what happens if nothing is done? *J Hypertens* 2005;23(suppl 3):S5–S13.

17. Mehta M, Darling RC, Roddy SP et al. Outcome of concomitant renal artery reconstructions in patients with aortic aneurysm and occlusive disease. *Vascular* 2004;12:381–6.

18. Senekowitsch C, Assadian A, Wlk MV et al. Renal artery surgery in the era of endovascular intervention. *Vasa* 2004;33:226–30.

19. Galaria II, Surowiec SM, Rhodes JM et al. Percutaneous and open renal revascularizations have equivalent outcomes. *Ann Vasc Surg* 2005;19:218–28.

20. Gray BH. Intervention for renal artery stenosis: endovascular and surgical roles. *J Hypertens* 2005;23(suppl 3):S23–9.

The role of the TASC classification in managing patients with aorto-iliac disease

André Nevelsteen MD PhD FRCS, Kim Daenens MD and Inge Fourneau MD PhD
Department of Vascular Surgery, University Hospital Gasthuisberg, Leuven, Belgium

In 2000, the TransAtlantic Inter-Society Consensus (TASC) Working Group published a historical document on the treatment of peripheral arterial disease (PAD).[1] This classified aorto-iliac disease into four categories based on severity (Figure 1), and recommended that minor lesions (TASC A) should be treated by endovascular means, and extensive lesions (TASC D) by open surgery. No consensus was reached on the treatment of 'intermediate lesions' (TASC B and C); more evidence was needed in order to recommend either endovascular techniques or open surgery for these. Over the last 5 years, great developments in both open surgery and, particularly, endovascular treatment have meant that the TASC document might be reconsidered. This issue was discussed at length in a multidisciplinary session between surgeons, interventionalists and radiologists at the Charing Cross Meeting in May 2005.

TASC A and TASC B lesions

A TASC A lesion comprises a single unilateral or bilateral stenosis of less than 3 cm in length in the common iliac or external iliac artery (Figure 1). A TASC B lesion comprises one of the following:
- a single stenosis 3–10 cm in length that does not extend into the common femoral artery
- a total of two stenoses less than 5 cm long in the common iliac and/or external iliac artery, but not extending into the common femoral artery
- a unilateral common iliac artery occlusion.

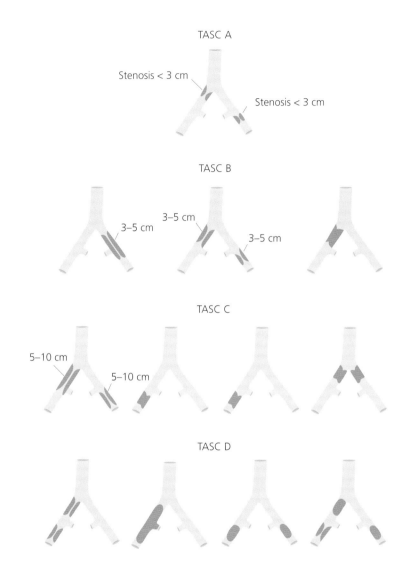

Figure 1 The TransAtlantic Inter-Society Consensus (TASC) classification of aorto-iliac lesions.

Management

Unilateral disease. It is agreed that endovascular intervention is the first treatment option. Its technical success rate in iliac artery stenosis has been reported to be 88–99% with a weighted average of 95%. For iliac occlusions, a success rate of 78–98% has been documented with a weighted average of 83%.[1] Open surgery is justified only after failure of endovascular intervention and, even then, the general condition of the patient, the disabling character of the symptoms and the distribution of the lesions should be taken into consideration before any decision is taken.

Bilateral disease. Although it is agreed that open surgery provides the best long-term results in bilateral disease, endovascular intervention remains the treatment of choice. When only one side is correctable by endovascular means, a major open operation might be avoided by unilateral endovascular therapy and femorofemoral bypass, which is considered as minor surgery and can be performed under regional or even local anesthesia.[2]

Endovascular reconstruction techniques. Despite the general agreement about the choice of endovascular treatment, the preferred technique for reconstruction or, more precisely, the need for stents in the iliac arteries, is still the subject of debate. Most interventionalists prefer stents for total occlusion,[3] but there is no evidence for primary stenting and certainly not in iliac stenosis. A randomized trial to compare simple balloon angioplasty and primary stenting has never been performed, and only one randomized trial to compare primary stenting and selective stenting has been reported. The Dutch Iliac Stent Trial (DIST) randomized 279 patients to either direct stent placement (n = 143) or primary angioplasty with subsequent stent placement if the residual pressure gradient was more than 10 mmHg (n = 136).[4] With 2-year cumulative patency rates of 71% and 70%, respectively, it was concluded that there were no substantial differences in the technical results and clinical outcomes in the two groups. Although this study showed that sequential stenting might be preferable, it did not demonstrate that stents are necessary. Nevertheless, despite the absence of firm evidence, primary and systematic stenting has become the rule rather than the exception in the day-to-day practice of most interventionalists.

There is also uncertainty about the results of endovascular treatment for external iliac artery disease. There are conflicting results in the literature, but some authors reported poor treatment outcomes for the external iliac artery compared with the common iliac artery.[5] The size of the iliac vessel has indeed been recognized as a risk factor in terms of long-term patency, which in turn might explain the relatively poor results in women.[6,7] In addition, in contrast to the case for the common iliac arteries, there are virtually no published data on external iliac artery occlusions.

TASC C and TASC D lesions

TASC C and TASC D aorto-iliac lesions include more extensive disease (Figure 1). A TASC C lesion comprises one of the following:
- bilateral 5–10 cm long stenosis of the common iliac artery and/or external iliac artery not involving the common femoral artery
- unilateral external iliac artery occlusion not involving the common femoral artery
- unilateral external iliac artery stenosis involving the common femoral artery
- bilateral common iliac artery occlusion.

TASC D lesions include:
- diffuse, multiple unilateral stenosis involving the common iliac artery, external iliac artery and common femoral artery
- unilateral occlusion of both common and external iliac arteries
- bilateral occlusion of the external iliac arteries
- diffuse disease involving the aorta and both iliac arteries
- iliac stenosis in a patient with an abdominal aortic aneurysm or other lesion requiring aortic or iliac surgery.

For TASC C and TASC D lesions, it is agreed that the long-term results of open surgery are far superior to those of endovascular treatment, and direct aorto-iliac reconstruction (aortobifemoral grafting) remains the treatment of choice.

Aortofemoral bypass is one of the few operations for which long-term results of up to 15 years postoperatively have been reported.[8] By 1997, de Vries and Hunink published a meta-analysis of 6000 patients from 23 studies in which they documented a primary patency rate at 5 and 10 years of 86% and 79%, respectively, following treatment for claudication compared with 82% and 72% for critical ischemia.[9]

These long-term results must, however, be balanced against the operative mortality and morbidity rates, which have been recognized as the major drawback of direct aorto-iliac reconstruction. Depending on the hospital and the patient's comorbidity, the operative mortality rate lies between 2% and 5%. As documented in the meta-analysis by de Vries and Hunink, although substantial improvement has been achieved over the years, even recent studies report a 3.3% mortality rate ($p = 0.01$ vs older studies).[9] The same is true for systemic morbidity, which decreased from 13.1% to 8.3% ($p < 0.001$). Further improvement might be expected from advances in perioperative medical treatment[10] and efforts to reduce surgical trauma. In this regard, enthusiasm for laparoscopic aortofemoral bypass is increasing. Coggia et al. published their experience with total laparoscopic bypass for TASC C and TASC D aorto-iliac lesions in 93 patients and concluded that laparoscopic techniques might reduce the operative trauma of aortic bypass.[11] Total laparoscopic bypass is, however, extremely technically demanding. As a result, hand-assisted laparoscopic aortofemoral bypass, which is technically less complex and produces midterm results comparable to those from open reconstruction, has been used as a tool to overcome the learning curve associated with total laparoscopic aorto-iliac surgery.[12] Currently, however, there is no firm evidence of the superiority of these laparoscopic techniques over traditional direct aorto-iliac grafting.

Femorofemoral bypass. Given the mortality and morbidity rates associated with direct aorto-iliac reconstruction, it is not surprising that, for several years, femorofemoral bypass has been suggested as an alternative, particularly for patients in whom open reconstruction poses a risk. With 5-year patency rates between 55% and 70%, it is certainly of proven value in unilateral disease. More recently, reports of the treatment of bilateral disease with unilateral endovascular reconstruction completed by crossover grafting have

Highlights in **the role of the TASC classification in managing patients with aorto-iliac disease** *2005–06*

WHAT'S IN?

- Endovascular treatment of TransAtlantic Inter-Society Consensus (TASC) A, TASC B and TASC C lesions
- Primary stenting for iliac occlusive disease
- Femorofemoral crossover graft for unilateral TASC D lesions
- Femorofemoral crossover bypass combined with endovascular techniques for bilateral TASC C and TASC D lesions
- Laparoscopic techniques for direct aortic reconstruction
- Optimization of preoperative medical therapy for direct aortic reconstruction

WHAT'S OUT?

- Open surgery for TASC A and TASC B lesions
- Conventional direct aorto-iliac bypass for TASC C and D lesions

WHAT'S NEEDED?

- A randomized study on the need of stents for iliac stenosis
- Contemporary data on the results of endovascular treatment of external iliac artery stenosis and occlusion
- Contemporary data on mortality, morbidity and quality of life after direct aorto-iliac bypass
- A randomized study on the treatment of bilateral TASC D lesions with direct bypass or crossover graft in combination with endovascular techniques
- A randomized study between laparoscopic and direct aorto-iliac bypass

also been encouraging.[2] In addition, there is evidence that crossover bypass is indeed a valid alternative to open reconstruction.

Three retrospective, non-randomized clinical studies that compared femorofemoral bypass with anatomical reconstruction showed no significant difference in long-term patency rates.[13–15] In 1997, Ricco et al. presented the only randomized trial comprising 143 patients, all of whom were of low surgical risk, which demonstrated no significant differences in operative mortality or morbidity rates; morbidity rate was 2.6% in the crossover group compared with 8.6% in the anatomical group ($p > 0.05$).[16] The 7-year primary patency rate was 86% in the anatomical group compared with 49% in the crossover group ($p = 0.006$). However, most of the failures in the crossover group were due to progression of disease in the donor iliac artery, and the 7-year secondary patency rates were 95% in the anatomical group and 79% in the crossover group ($p = 0.08$). It was concluded that a direct bypass procedure achieves the best long-term results at the cost of a moderate increase in operative morbidity.

References

1. Dormandy JA, Rutherford RB. Management of peripheral arterial disease (PAD). TASC Working Group. TransAtlantic Inter-Society Consensus (TASC). *Eur J Vasc Endovasc Surg* 2000;19(suppl A): S1–244; *J Vasc Surg* 2000;31: S1–296.

2. Aburhama AF, Robinson PA, Cook CC, Hopkins ES. Selecting patients for combined femorofemoral bypass grafting and iliac balloon angioplasty and stenting for bilateral iliac disease. *J Vasc Surg* 2001;33(2 suppl):S93–9.

3. Bosch JL, Tetteroo E, Mali WP, Hunink MG. Iliac arterial occlusive disease: cost-effectiveness analysis of stent placement versus percutaneous transluminal angioplasty. *Radiology* 1998;208:641–8.

4. Tetteroo E, van der Graaf Y, Bosch JL et al. Randomised comparison of primary stent placement versus primary angioplasty followed by selective stent placement in patients with iliac-artery occlusive disease. Dutch Iliac Stent Trial Study Group. *Lancet* 1998;351:1153–9.

5. Murphy TP, Ariaratnam NS, Carney WI Jr et al. Aortoiliac insufficiency: long-term experience with stent placement for treatment. *Radiology* 2004;231:243–9.

6. Carnevale FC, De Blas M, Merino S et al. Percutaneous endovascular treatment of chronic iliac artery occlusion. *Cardiovasc Intervent Radiol* 2004;27:447–52.

7. Timaran CH, Stevens SL, Freeman MB, Goldman MH. External iliac and common iliac artery angioplasty and stenting in men and women. *J Vasc Surg* 2001;34:440–6.

8. Nevelsteen A, Wouters L, Suy R. Aortofemoral Dacron reconstruction for aortoiliac occlusive disease: a 25-year survey. *Eur J Vasc Surg* 1991;5:179–86.

9. de Vries SO, Hunink MG. Results of aortic bifurcation grafts for aortoiliac occlusive disease: a meta-analysis. *J Vasc Surg* 1997;26:558–69.

10. Poldermans D, Boersma E, Bax JJ et al. Bisoprolol reduces cardiac death and myocardial infarction in high-risk patients as long as 2 years after successful major vascular surgery. *Eur Heart J* 2001;22:1253–5.

11. Coggia M, Javerliat I, Di Centa I et al. Total laparoscopic bypass for aortoiliac occlusive lesions: 93-case experience. *J Vasc Surg* 2004;40:899–906.

12. Fourneau I, Daenens K, Nevelsteen A. Hand-assisted laparoscopic aortobifemoral bypass for occlusive disease. Early and midterm results. *Eur J Vasc Endovasc Surg* 2005;30:489–93.

13. Lorenzi G, Domanin M, Costantini A et al. Role of bypass, endarterectomy, extra-anatomic bypass and endovascular surgery in unilateral iliac occlusive disease: a review of 1257 cases. *Cardiovasc Surg* 1994;2:370–3.

14. Nazzal MM, Hoballah JJ, Jacobovicz C et al. A comparative evaluation of femorofemoral crossover bypass with iliofemoral bypass for unilateral iliac artery occlusive disease. *Angiology* 1998;49:259–65.

15. Mingoli A, Sapienza P, Feldhaus RJ et al. Comparison of femorofemoral and aortofemoral bypass for aortoiliac occlusive disease. *J Cardiovasc Surg* 2001;42:381–7.

16. AURC and Ricco JB, Bouin-Pineau MH, Demarque C et al. Late results after femorofemoral crossover bypass surgery. A randomised study. In: Branchereau A, Jacobs M, eds. *Long-term results of arterial interventions.* New York: Futura Publications, 1997:15–166.

The role of the TASC classification in managing patients with infra-inguinal arterial disease

Peter R Taylor MA MChir FRCS and Tom WG Carrell MA MChir FRCS

Guy's & St. Thomas' NHS Foundation Trust, London, UK

The TransAtlantic Inter-Society Consensus (TASC) classification of patients presenting with infra-inguinal disease describes four categories of femoropopliteal lesions (Table 1).[1] The recommendations suggested by the TASC group in 2000 were that TASC A femoropopliteal lesions should be treated by percutaneous transluminal angioplasty and that TASC D required surgical bypass. No recommendation was made for TASC B and C lesions, as evidence to support any particular intervention was lacking.

Further treatment options have become available since the publication of the TASC document; these include debulking devices,

TABLE 1

TransAtlantic Inter-Society Consensus classification of femoropopliteal lesions[1]

Category A	Single stenosis less than 3 cm long in the superficial femoral artery
Category B	Single stenosis or occlusion 3–5 cm long or multiple stenoses less than 3 cm long
Category C	Single stenosis or occlusion over 5 cm long, or multiple stenoses or occlusions each 3–5 cm long
Category D	Occlusion of the common or superficial femoral arteries, or popliteal and proximal trifurcation

cryoplasty, laser angioplasty, bare and covered stents, and dissolvable stents. In addition, improvements in non-invasive imaging, such as computerized tomographic angiography and magnetic resonance angiography combined with duplex ultrasonography, mean that lesions can be classified accurately before arterial puncture is performed, which enables more detailed forward planning of endoluminal interventions.

The TASC classification can provide a useful means of stratifying the severity of lesions in clinical studies. These results must, however, be interpreted cautiously in light of the presenting symptoms, comorbidity and the presence of significant inflow or outflow disease.

More widespread use of the classification in clinical publications and in clinical audit may help to clarify the indications for the diverse infra-inguinal interventions available, and enable individual clinicians to compare their own results with other centers.

Problems in assessing the TASC classification

Relatively few randomized, prospective trials of infra-inguinal interventions have been conducted, and most have had low statistical power with a short duration follow-up, often only 6–12 months. There are often mixed indications for intervention, and no distinction is made between patients with critical limb ischemia and those with claudication. Similarly, patients with diabetes and renal failure, who have a poor outcome, are usually included in these studies. Critical ischemia, diabetes and renal failure are also generally associated with poor distal run-off, which carries a higher risk of interventional failure than does claudication with good distal run-off. Interpretation of these studies can be further complicated by studies that mix primary, primary-assisted and even secondary patency as endpoint measures.

A Medline search reveals very few publications that address the effectiveness of the TASC classification in predicting the success of femoropopliteal intervention. This is partly because of the difficulty in performing such randomized controlled trials, but is also because of the short time that the TASC classification has been in print.

Balloon angioplasty and stent placement

The forces acting on the superficial femoral artery are complex and include extension, compression, rotation, yawing and bending. These forces, combined with low flow velocities, make the superficial femoral artery one of the most hostile environments in the body for the placement of metallic stents. High rates of early restenosis, occlusion and stent fracture are seen compared with those for the iliac and coronary vessels.

A recent large, retrospective study based on the TASC classification has evaluated the results of intervention in 329 patients in a single center over a 16-year period.[2] Most patients had claudication (66%) and the rest had critical limb ischemia. Most patients underwent angioplasty alone (63%) and, in 7% of patients, the lesion could not be crossed. The lesions were classified as 48% TASC A, 18% TASC B, 22% TASC C and 12% TASC D. Primary patency rates were heavily dependent on the TASC classification, with TASC A performing the best and TASC D the worst. The report concluded that TASC A and B lesions do as well with angioplasty as with surgery, but TASC C and D lesions do better with surgery.

A small study from Marseille examined the outcomes over 3 years in 32 patients (15 with claudication and 17 with critical or acute ischemia) treated with covered stents.[3] TASC D lesions were excluded. Simultaneous outflow procedures were performed in 12 of the 15 patients with critical ischemia. The results showed 81% primary patency rates for the claudication group and 87% for the critical/acute ischemia group at 12 months. The authors state that patients with critical or acute limb ischemia can have as good an outcome as claudicants with good run-off, if concomitant procedures to improve outflow are performed.

There is some evidence that primary uncovered stents have poorer patency rates than primary angioplasty with selective stenting,[4] and the effectiveness of this policy was examined in a retrospective review of 115 TASC B femoropopliteal lesions.[5] The study concluded that endovascular therapy for TASC B lesions was safe, but both selective stenting and angioplasty alone were associated with a risk of recurrent stenosis at 1 year. Of those who had a stent, 49% had developed a restenosis, compared with 42% of those who underwent angioplasty alone, although this difference was not statistically significant.

Almost by definition, TASC D lesions are the least favorable for endovascular intervention and this is echoed in a retrospective analysis of 441 femoropopliteal lesions,[6] which showed that TASC D lesions and critical ischemia were the strongest predictors of early failure. The TASC classification has also been used to stratify lesions in the crural segment and, unsurprisingly, the worst results for transluminal angioplasty in these vessels is seen with the more complex TASC C and D lesions.[7]

Debulking procedures

The poor long-term results of angioplasty and stenting to treat long and multiple lesions in the femoropopliteal segment has led to continued interest in other means of dealing with these lesions. Debulking procedures rely on removing atheromatous plaque rather than compression in angioplasty.

A 60% primary patency at 18 months has been reported with the use of remote superficial femoral artery endarterectomy of TASC D lesions in 56 claudicants and 6 patients with critical ischemia.[8] These results are comparable with surgical bypass, but the general applicability of the technique appears to be limited by the requirement for a suitable end-zone below the treated segment. A stent may be required to tack down the distal extent of the atherectomy. Similar results have been reported in a separate multicenter trial in the USA.[9]

Minimally invasive atherectomy using a mechanical device (SilverHawk) has been reported to result in a 27% restenosis rate at 6 months for primary TASC A to C femoropopliteal stenoses (1–30 cm, no occlusions), although the long-term results remain unknown.[10] Successful recanalization of long superficial femoral artery occlusions (TASC D) has been reported in 85% of cases treated by excimer percutaneous transluminal

Highlights in the role of the TASC classification in managing patients with infra-inguinal arterial disease 2005–06

WHAT'S IN?

- Non-invasive imaging, such as computerized tomographic angiography or magnetic resonance angiography, to plan percutaneous interventions

- Transluminal angioplasty for TransAtlantic Inter-Society Consensus (TASC) A and B lesions

WHAT'S OUT?

- Routine diagnostic intra-arterial arteriography

- Publication of small studies with mixed indications and short-term follow-up

WHAT'S CONTROVERSIAL?

- Debulking procedures, such as remote superficial femoral endarterectomy, mechanical atherectomy and laser angioplasty

- The role of covered stents in TASC C and D lesions

laser angioplasty, although reservations remain because of the 28% 4-year primary patency and the high capital cost of the laser.[11]

References

1. Dormandy JA, Rutherford RB. Management of peripheral arterial disease (PAD). TASC Working Group. TransAtlantic Inter-Society Consensus (TASC). *J Vasc Surg* 2000;31:S1–296.

2. Surowiec SM, Davies MG, Eberly SW et al. Percutaneous angioplasty and stenting of the superficial femoral artery. *J Vasc Surg* 2005;41:269–78.

3. Hartung O, Otero A, Dubuc M et al. Efficacy of Hemobahn in the treatment of superficial femoral artery lesions in patients with acute or critical ischemia: a comparative study with claudicants. *Eur J Vasc Endovasc Surg* 2005:30:300–6.

4. Becquemin JP, Favre JP, Marzelle J et al. Systematic versus selective stent placement after superficial femoral balloon angioplasty: a multicenter prospective randomized study. *J Vasc Surg* 2003;37:487–94.

5. Costanza MJ, Queral LA, Lilly MP, Finn WR. Hemodynamic outcome of endovascular therapy for TransAtlantic InterSociety Consensus type B femoropopliteal arterial occlusive lesions. *J Vasc Surg* 2004;39:343–50.

6. Galaria II, Surowiec SM, Rhodes JM et al. Implications of early failure of superficial femoral artery endoluminal interventions. *Ann Vasc Surg* 2005;19:787–92.

7. Sigala F, Menenakos Ch, Sigalas P et al. Transluminal angioplasty of isolated crural arterial lesions in diabetics with critical limb ischemia. *Vasa* 2005;34:186–91.

8. Knight JS, Smeets L, Morris GE, Moll FL. Multi centre study to assess the feasibility of a new covered stent and delivery system in combination with remote superficial femoral artery endarterectomy (RSFAE). *Eur J Vasc Endovasc Surg* 2005;29:287–94.

9. Rosenthal D, Martin JD, Schubart PJ et al. Remote superficial femoral artery endarterectomy and distal aspire stenting: multicenter medium-term results. *J Vasc Surg* 2004;40:67–72.

10. Zeller T, Rastan A, Schwarzwalder U et al. Percutaneous peripheral atherectomy of femoropopliteal stenoses using a new-generation device: six-month results from a single-center experience. *J Endovasc Ther* 2004;11:676–85.

11. Wissgott C, Scheinert D, Rademaker J et al. Treatment of long superficial femoral artery occlusions with excimer laser angioplasty: long-term results after 48 months. *Acta Radiol* 2004;45:23–9.

Treatment options for iliofemoral vein thrombosis

Jürg Schmidli MD and Georg Heller MD

Department of Cardiovascular Surgery, University Hospital, Bern, Switzerland

It has been estimated that the yearly incidence of acute deep-vein thrombosis (DVT) is about 250 000 cases in the USA alone.[1] Among the potential sequelae of a DVT is postthrombotic syndrome (PTS), which includes chronic pain, edema and ulceration. About 50% of patients with proximal DVT will develop PTS within 1 year.[2] The long-term consequences are seldom documented. Most authors describe the resolution of the thrombus and (partial) recanalization,[3] although the goal of treatment should be prevention of the reflux that occurs in 96% after 5 years in conservative therapy;[4] this prevention can be achieved with intact venous valves only. The ideal therapy consists of the complete restoration of the venous lumen, preservation of vein valve function, prevention of pulmonary embolism and prevention of PTS.

Treatment options

Conservative treatment

Anticoagulation. The standard of care for DVT treatment is unfractionated heparin (UFH) and its derivatives, which include low-molecular-weight heparin (LMWH) and pentasaccharides. The incidence of heparin-induced thrombocytopenia (HIT) is 10 times lower with LMWH than with UFH. The pentasaccharides, including fondaparinux, have not been associated with HIT. Subcutaneous administration allows for outpatient therapy, and routine coagulation monitoring is not required. Although these drugs are relatively new for DVT treatment, they may offer certain advantages.[5]

Anticoagulation with LMWH is usually followed by a course of a vitamin K antagonist lasting from 3 months to a lifetime. As a long-term anticoagulant vitamin K antagonist, coumadin has been the standard of care for decades. The disadvantages of vitamin K antagonists are numerous, including the need for constant and continuous patient monitoring and the fact that major bleeding occurs in up to 10% of patients. New drugs may improve care in patients requiring chronic anticoagulation.[6]

Thrombolytic treatment makes it possible to eliminate the thrombus from the obstructed vein segments in DVT and to reduce the chance of subsequent reflux and venous hypertension damage. Thrombolytic agents can be administered systemically, locoregionally into a foot vein, catheter-directed into the thrombus or by means of a fragmentation device. The general disadvantage is the long duration of the procedure[7] and the high dosage of thrombolytic agents, which can easily lead to complications.[8]

Systemic thrombolysis. Thrombolysis of acute DVT less than 5 days old has had a higher success rate than in patients with old clots. Many studies have been completed comparing different thrombolytic agents with anticoagulant treatment, demonstrating improved patency rates and venous valvular competence for the former. Nevertheless, major bleeding complications can be as high as 11%; minor bleeding complications occur in 16% of patients, and pulmonary embolism and death must be taken into account too.[9,10]

Interventional treatment

Thrombectomy devices. In recent years, percutaneous motorized thrombectomy devices have been introduced. There are two categories:
- rotational devices
- hydrodynamic devices.

Rotational thrombectomy devices use a high-speed rotating basket or impeller to fragment the thrombus. The resultant small particles usually travel to the pulmonary circulation. In hydrodynamic devices the thrombus is fragmented by a jet and the particles are then aspirated into the device. One device, which combines a high

Highlights in **treatment options for iliofemoral vein thrombosis** *2005–06*

WHAT'S IN?

- Combined regional thrombolysis and surgical thrombectomy
- Percutaneous hydrodynamic devices in the iliofemoral axis
- Adjunct procedures of the common iliac vein (angioplasty/stenting) to secure outflow

WHAT'S OUT?

- Surgical thrombectomy of valve containing veins
- High-speed fragmentation devices in valve-containing veins
- Systemic thrombolytic therapy
- Conventional anticoagulation therapy only for acute iliofemoral DVT

WHAT'S CONTROVERSIAL?

- Catheter-directed thrombolysis

WHAT'S NEEDED?

- Randomized clinical controlled trial of combined regional thrombolysis and surgical thrombectomy versus standard anticoagulation therapy
- Randomized clinical controlled trial of interventional treatment versus standard anticoagulation therapy

concentration of thrombolytic agent with mechanical disruption of the clot, has been used with some success for rapid thrombus removal in patients with DVT.[11] Although promising, experience with these devices is still limited, and there are few published studies documenting their usefulness in patients with acute DVT.

Surgical thrombectomy. Enthusiasm for surgical thrombectomy in patients with DVT has fallen among physicians in many countries due to poor results. Only Plate et al. managed to describe a series of surgical thrombectomy in acute iliofemoral DVT. Iliac vein patency was 83% in surgical patients compared with 41% of patients receiving anticoagulation therapy. Venous physiological function and postthrombotic symptoms were both worse in the anticoagulation group.[12] However, surgical thrombectomy can only be successful in patients with proximal iliofemoral DVT without involvement of the deep venous valves.

Combined regional thrombolysis and surgical thrombectomy.
The thrombolytic agent is administered through a foot vein and a tourniquet is placed on the thigh. The drug is allowed to react for 30 minutes. Through a groin incision the femoral and iliac vein axis is cleared by means of a Fogarty catheter under general anesthesia. Then the cuff is removed and the thrombus flushed out from the leg veins. With this procedure vein patency and valve function were restored in 100% of a series of 33 patients. No major bleeding, pulmonary embolism or death occurred. At 6 to 10 years there was no postthrombotic syndrome.[13]

References

1. Augustinos P, Ouriel K. Invasive approaches to treatment of venous thromboembolism. *Circulation* 2004;110(9 suppl 1):I27–34.

2. Lopez-Azkarreta I, Reus S, Marco P et al. Prospective study of the risk factors for the development of post-thrombotic syndrome after proximal deep venous thrombosis [Spanish]. *Med Clin (Barc)* 2005;125:1–4.

3. Yamaki T, Nozaki M. Patterns of venous insufficiency after an acute deep vein thrombosis. *J Am Coll Surg* 2005;201:231–8.

4. Asbeutah AM, Riha AZ, Cameron JD, McGrath BP. Five-year outcome study of deep vein thrombosis in the lower limbs. *J Vasc Surg* 2004;40:1184–9.

5. Hyers TM. Heparin and other rapidly acting anticoagulants. *Semin Vasc Surg* 2005;18:130–3.

6. Ansell J. Long-term anticoagulation: the prospects for alternatives to warfarin. *Semin Vasc Surg* 2005;18:134–8.

7. Sillesen H, Just S, Jorgensen M, Baekgaard N. Catheter directed thrombolysis for treatment of ilio-femoral deep venous thrombosis is durable, preserves venous valve function and may prevent chronic venous insufficiency. *Eur J Vasc Endovasc Surg* 2005;30:556–62.

8. Schweizer J, Kirch W, Koch R et al. Short- and long-term results after thrombolytic treatment of deep venous thrombosis. *J Am Coll Cardiol* 2000;36:1336–43.

9. Mewissen MW. Catheter-directed thrombolysis for lower extremity deep vein thrombosis. *Tech Vasc Interv Radiol* 2001;4:111–14.

10. Mewissen MW, Saebrook GR, Meissner MH et al. Catheter-directed thrombolysis for lower extremity deep venous thrombosis: report of a national multicenter registry. *Radiology* 1999;211:39–49.

11. Ramaiah V, Del Santo PB, Rodriguez-Lopez JA et al. Trellis thrombectomy system for the treatment of iliofemoral deep venous thrombosis. *J Endovasc Ther* 2003;10:585–9.

12. Plate G, Eklof B, Norgren L et al. Venous thrombectomy for iliofemoral vein thrombosis – 10-year results of a prospective randomized study. *Eur J Vasc Endovasc Surg* 1997;14:367–74.

13. Blattler W, Heller G, Largiader J et al. Combined regional thrombolysis and surgical thrombectomy for treatment of iliofemoral vein thrombosis. *J Vasc Surg* 2004;40:620–5.

Foam sclerotherapy vs laser/radio-frequency ablation for management of great saphenous vein incompetence

Nick Morrison MD FACS FACPh

Morrison Vein Institute, Scottsdale, Arizona, USA

Management of great saphenous vein incompetence has historically been treated with flush ligation of the great saphenous vein at the saphenofemoral junction, ligation of all tributaries, and groin-to-ankle or groin-to-knee stripping of the saphenous vein.[1] Since 1999, first radiofrequency (RF) and then laser endovenous thermal ablation procedures, and more recently endovenous chemical ablation procedures, have been found to be safe and effective methods of eliminating the proximal portion of the great saphenous vein from the venous circulation, with faster recovery and better cosmetic results than stripping.[2-4] The thermal ablation systems use electromagnetic energy to destroy the proximal great saphenous vein; chemical ablation utilizes a foamed detergent (commonly Polidocanol or sodium tetradecylsulfate). As with a stripping procedure, following these endovenous ablation procedures it is necessary to treat any remaining portion of the great and/or small saphenous vein, perforator veins, and tributaries additionally with either injection sclerotherapy and/or phlebectomy.[5]

Patient selection

Inclusion criteria are: symptoms and physical signs of venous insufficiency; duplex scan, performed by a fully qualified sonographer, demonstrating a patent great saphenous vein with reflux longer than 0.5 s; patent deep venous system; vein conducive to catheterization or injection; and full patient mobility. Absolute exclusion criteria are: arteriovenous malformations; restricted ambulation; and deep venous obstruction. As a practitioner's experience with thermal endovenous ablation procedures expands, relative exclusion criteria may be relaxed, so patients with partial sclerosis from previous venous treatment, large diameter veins, or those receiving chronic anticoagulant therapy or hormone replacement therapy may be safely and successfully treated. These relative exclusion criteria do not generally apply to endovenous chemical ablation.

Procedures

Details of the thermal ablation procedures can be found in various reports[6,7] and will not be reiterated in detail here. The differences in technique between thermal and chemical endovenous ablation are few but significant.

The RF catheter or laser fiber is inserted into the saphenous vein using the Seldinger technique. Access to the great saphenous vein for chemical ablation can be accomplished either with direct needle access or with a catheter inserted into the great saphenous vein. Saphenofemoral occlusion, either by external compression or with a balloon-tipped catheter, permits retention of foamed sclerosant in the vein long enough to produce adequate damage to cause sclerosis.

Generally, both thermal ablation techniques utilize dilute local anesthetic injected into the saphenous sheath under ultrasound guidance. This step is not necessary with chemical ablation.

Procedural costs are highest for RF ablation, somewhat less for laser ablation, and significantly lower for chemical ablation.

Complications

Intraoperative and postoperative complications occur infrequently, and are generally well tolerated and short-lived.[2,4,8] Intraoperative complications with thermal ablation techniques include: difficult device access or advancement; treatment interruption (RF only); and transient heat. Postoperatively patients may encounter bruising and pain (more often with laser); paresthesia; thermal skin damage; superficial thrombophlebitis; and lymphedema.[9] Deep-vein thrombosis, the most clinically significant complication, may occur after any endovenous ablation procedure.[9] The risk is generally reported to be less than 1%,[3,4,10] usually involving calf veins.

Side effects only seen following foam chemical ablation include dry cough, chest discomfort, nausea, visual disturbances, headache, dizziness, and psychogenic reactions.[11] They are infrequent, and usually resolve spontaneously within 24 hours. Except for dry cough, these reactions are not related to volume of foam injected. In a recent study, 7 patients with these post-foam symptoms and a patent foramen ovale (proven on bubble study) had simultaneous peripheral foam sclerotherapy, transthoracic echocardiography, and transcranial Doppler ultrasonography.[12] Bubbles were identified in the left heart within 10 s of the initial 1 cm^3 foam injection in all patients, and emboli were identified in the middle cerebral artery in 4 of 7. The relationship of the emboli to patients' symptoms is unclear at this time, but it is of some concern.

One complication of great interest because of its relative absence following endovenous ablation is neovascularization.[6] Neovascularization is commonly seen following the traditional ligation/stripping procedure,[5] and is thought to be secondary to 'frustrated' venous drainage from the abdominal wall and perineum. Whether this is actually the development of new veins, or simply enlargement of previously existing veins, the result is recurrent reflux in thigh or lower leg veins. Endovenous ablation of the great saphenous vein deliberately leaves the superficial epigastric vein intact, which, it is believed, has resulted in few reports of neovascularization.[6]

Results

Early reports from 1999–2000, and follow-up reports as long as 5 years after RF ablation confirm the safety and efficacy of this method of saphenous vein ablation.[6,10,13] Successful ablation rates of 85% or more are routinely demonstrated.[14]

In a prospective randomized study directly comparing RF ablation with stripping, Lurie et al. demonstrated excellent success rates for RF ablation comparable to or better than those following stripping.[15]

Following the introduction of RF ablation of the great saphenous vein, reports from some centers were published, beginning in 2000–2001, which appeared to show an unprecedented rate of successful ablation (100%) of the great saphenous vein using laser energy, with few or no complications.[16] Follow-up data over 3 years appear to confirm earlier high success rates.[7,8] Other centers, including that of Proebstle, also report high rates of successful ablation using lasers of various wavelengths.[3]

Numerous reports from Europe, including from Frullini[4] and Cavezzi,[17] have demonstrated excellent results of endovenous ablation of the truncal veins with foamed chemical detergent sclerosants, including Polidocanol and sodium tetradecylsulfate.

Discussion

Much confusion exists in the literature regarding the definition of successful treatment, the means used to detect treatment failures and the reporting of results. Recent advances in the technology of ultrasound have resulted in more critical evaluation of clinical results than were possible in the past. Duplex examination for successful ablation of a vein should include grayscale, compression and color flow Doppler. Identification of treatment failure depends on the sensitivity of the ultrasound equipment used for postoperative examination, the expertise of the sonographer and the vigor with which the examination is conducted.

Foam sclerotherapy has had an unexpected effect on critical analysis of successful ablation. Because foam is an excellent contrast medium with ultrasound, injection of foam into distal vein segments, tributaries and incompetent perforators will sometimes reveal an incompletely treated vein that appears completely occluded by all other duplex ultrasound criteria. This further calls into question even the most critical examination techniques. Whether these minimally patent segments will become clinically significant is unanswered at present, but certainly patients who complain of localized pain in the area of a previously ablated vein deserve very careful examination to identify the incompletely ablated segment.

Highlights in **foam sclerotherapy vs laser/radiofrequency ablation for management of great saphenous vein incompetence** 2005–06

WHAT'S IN?

- Ablation of the great saphenous vein with:
  - foam chemical ablation
  - laser thermal ablation
  - radiofrequency thermal ablation

WHAT'S OUT?

- Traditional groin-to-ankle stripping

WHAT'S NEEDED?

- Careful follow-up by duplex ultrasonography
- Uniform definitions of 'successful' ablation
- Long-term data
- Further information regarding bubble emboli

Because of the risk of incomplete ablation or recurrent patency of the treated vein, and the need for adjunctive treatment of the distal great saphenous vein, the refluxing tributaries and small saphenous vein, interval color flow Doppler ultrasound, interviews and physical examinations are necessary to achieve successful treatment. It is not enough merely to ablate the proximal vein and expect the patient's symptoms and varicosities to resolve. Unless one is committed to careful follow-up and adjunctive treatment, the patient and the practitioner will be left with unsatisfactory results.

References

1. Sarin S, Scurr JH, Coleridge-Smith PD. Stripping of the long saphenous vein in the treatment of primary varicose veins. *Br J Surg* 1994;81:1455–8.

2. Kistner RL. Endovascular obliteration of the greater saphenous vein: the closure procedure. *Jpn J Phlebol* 2002;13:325–33.

3. Proebstle TM, Gül D, Lehr HA et al. Infrequent early recanalization of greater saphenous vein after endovenous laser treatment. *J Vasc Surg* 2003;38:511–16.

4. Frullini A, Cavezzi A. Sclerosing foam in the treatment of varicose veins and telangiectases: history and analysis of safety and complications. *Derm Surg* 2002;28:11–15.

5. Fischer R, Chandler JG, De Maeseneer MG et al. The unresolved problem of recurrent saphenofemoral reflux. *J Am Coll Surg* 2002;195:80–94.

6. Pichot O, Kabnick LS, Creton D et al. Duplex ultrasound scan findings two years after great saphenous vein radiofrequency endovenous obliteration. *J Vasc Surg* 2004;39:189–95.

7. Navarro L, Min RJ, Bone C. Endovenous laser: a new minimally invasive treatment for varicose veins – preliminary observations using an 810 nm diode laser. *Derm Surg* 2001;27:117–22.

8. Min RJ, Khilnani N, Zimmer S. Endovenous laser treatment of saphenous vein reflux: long-term results. *J Vasc Surg* 2003;14:991–6.

9. Morrison N. Comparative study of radiofrequency vs laser ablation of the greater saphenous vein. Unpublished data presented at *Liverpool Endovascular Masterclass*, Liverpool, UK: 17 October 2004.

10. Weiss RA, Weiss MA. Controlled radiofrequency endovenous occlusion using a unique radiofrequency catheter under duplex guidance to eliminate saphenous varicose vein reflux: A 2-year follow-up. *Dermatol Surg* 2002;28:38–42.

11. Morrison N. Large-volume, ultrasound-guided, polidocanol foam sclerotherapy: a prospective study of toxicity and complications. Presented at *Union Internationale de Phlebologie*, San Diego, USA: September 2003.

12. Morrison N. Simultaneous ultrasound-guided sclerotherapy, transthoracic echocardiography and transcranial doppler. Presented at *Union Internationale de Phlebologie*, Rio de Janeiro, Brazil: October 2005.

13. Merchant RF, Pichot O. Long-term outcomes of endovenous radiofrequency obliteration of saphenous reflux as a treatment for superficial venous insufficiency. *J Vasc Surg* 2005;42:502–9.

14. Nicolini P; Closure Group. Treatment of primary varicose veins by endovenous obliteration with the VNUS closure system: results of a prospective multicentre study. *Eur J Vasc Endovasc Surg* 2005;29:433–9.

15. Lurie F, Creton D, Eklof B et al. Prospective randomised study of endovenous radiofrequency obliteration (closure) versus ligation and vein stripping (EVOLVeS): Two-year follow-up. *Eur J Vasc Endovasc Surg* 2005;29:67–73.

16. Min RJ, Zimmet SE, Isaacs MN, Forrestal MD. Endovenous laser treatment of the incompetent greater saphenous vein. *J Vasc Interv Radiol* 2001;12:1167–71.

17. Cavezzi A, Frullini A, Ricci S, Tessari L. Treatment of varicose veins by foam sclerotherapy: two clinical series. *Phlebology* 2002;17:13–18.

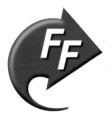

Imagine if every time
you wanted to know something
you knew where to look...

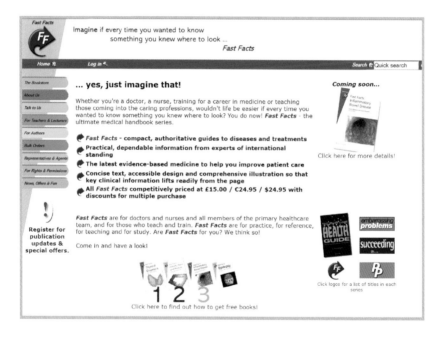

... **you do now!**

www.fastfacts.com